OPERATION OPTIMAL

HEALTH, WELLNESS, AND BECOMING YOUR BEST YOU

TOMO MARJANOVIC

tomomarjanovic.com

Cover design by Kristen Andrews
Interior Design by Heidi Sutherlin
Author photography by Gary Rice

Printed in the United States of America.

ISBNs

979-8-9957151-0-8 (Paperback)
979-8-9957151-1-5 (Hardcover)
979-8-9957151-2-2 (eBook)
979-8-9957151-3-9 (Audiobook)

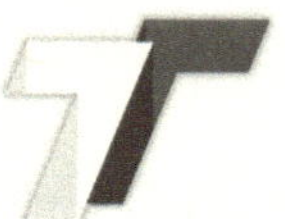

Tomo LLC
8014 Via Dellagio Way #201A, Orlando, FL 32819

CONTENTS

INTRODUCTION

Nobody's coming to save you.

Not your doctor. Not the medical system. Not some miracle drug or next-generation treatment. If you want to be healthy, *truly healthy*, it's on you. It's your responsibility. And honestly? It's your fault if you're not.

I know that sounds harsh, but it's the truth. And the truth is beautiful once you understand it. Because if your health is your responsibility, that means you have the power to change it right now.

Today.

I learned this lesson young. When I was 12 or 13, I grew so fast one summer in Croatia that my body couldn't keep up. Extreme joint pain. Stretch marks on my lower back from growing too tall too quickly. I left as one of the shorter kids in my friend group and came back the tallest, in three months. The doctor told me the only solution was to strengthen the muscles around my joints.

No pills.

No shortcuts.

Just hard work.

That sent me down a path I'm still on today. From that

moment, I understood that optimization was the goal. Being "normal" isn't good enough. In fact, being normal today means being overweight, on multiple medications, and chronically sick. That's the average. That's what happens when you follow the standard American lifestyle.

But here's what most people don't realize: getting healthy is simple. The recipe is easy: Stop eating fast food. Stop drinking soda. Go for walks. Those three things alone could change your entire life. The difficulty is in doing the work.

This book isn't about complicated protocols or expensive treatments. It's about taking responsibility. It's about understanding that the more muscle you have, the longer you'll live. That your gut health affects your brain. That your physical body and mental health are completely tied together. These aren't theories but verified medical science.

If you just start—if you make one small change and take responsibility for your own health—you'll go down a rabbit hole that transforms you completely. Just give five percent effort to start. Just change one habit. Then another. That's how you become someone unrecognizable from who you are today.

So let me be clear: This book is your wake-up call. Nobody cares about your health except you. Once you accept that, once you get past that hurdle and start taking baby steps, everything changes.

Welcome to *Operation Optimal*. Let's get to work.

—Tomo Marjanovic

PART I

CHAPTER 1

Own Your Own Health

Our health is failing us because our healthcare has betrayed it.

Big Pharma and Big Medicine celebrate our symptom suppression as *success*; normalizes our chronic fatigue as *adulthood*; and mistakes our over-medication for medicine. Behind their sterile masks of "standards of care" lies a machine designed to keep us dependent, docile, and just alive enough to pay for more. For them, "a patient cured is a patient lost."

We live in the greatest chronic illness crisis the world has ever seen, and modern medicine's answer is *pills before progress*. It's like patching the Titanic with chewing gum. To stop the sinking, we must first ask the question: *why is the ship going down in the first place?*

I'm Tomo Marjanovic. I've spent my life in the service of others, first as a police officer and now as an entrepreneur in healthcare innovation. If there's one lesson which I've learned through all of that, it's this:

Own your own health.

Because if you don't, someone else will.

Most people today are in the exact opposite mindset of that. When they get sick or chronically ill, they don't question why. Rather, they say, "I'll go right to my doctor. They'll send me to a specialist. The specialist will tell me to take this pill or undergo that procedure, and that'll get me fixed."

That sounds like the normal response… Well, the *normal* often falls far short of the *optimal* nowadays. We have gotten used to the second-rate. We blindly trust authority and funnel ourselves into a system that I call **a pill for every ill**, a system that addresses symptoms and not the root causes of our chronic illnesses.

Isn't there *a better way*?

I hope to show you that there is. This book is about **empowering you** to go on your own health journey without Big Pharma, Big Medicine, or mainstream doctors *dictating* how it's going to be without your say in the process. It's your body, and *you* should be the expert on it, not someone else!

So, with that in mind, let's get started.

A LITTLE BIT ABOUT ME

I'm a first generation American. I was born into a family of Croatian immigrants, who came to the US pursuing the American Dream (which has come true for us by the way). But when I was 12 years old, something very strange happened that changed my mindset about health and wellness forever.

I took a trip to Europe with my father for the summer. I had a massive growth spurt over there. I grew six or seven inches and came back with intense growth pains. I had side-way stretch marks on my lower back and knees. I went in to the doctor to see what could be done about my pain.

Do you know what my doctor prescribed?

Weightlifting!

It was the best prescription I've ever received. He said the best thing to do was to strengthen my muscles around my joints. That's how I first got into the gym.

This was the 90s. I grew up in that era where muscles were the big thing: Schwarzenegger, Jean-Claude Van Damme, Stallone. All the action stars back then were *jacked*. One day, I was watching the documentary "Pumping Iron", and it all clicked for me. I realized that weightlifting and bodybuilding, strengthening your muscles, wasn't just a sport; it was a crucial part of health – body, mind, and spirit.

I decided to follow my doctor's advice. Instead of *treating* my pain by taking painkillers, I committed to *strengthening* my body. I was ambitious. When I was 19, I told my coach I wanted to be Mr. Olympia. I wanted to take steroids. My coach laughed and told me to get my labs done first!

That's how my journey into bodybuilding, fitness modeling, and studying anti-aging, hormones, and wellness began. Little did I know it then, this decision would save and change my life one day.

WHAT BEING A COP TAUGHT ME ABOUT HEALTH

I became a cop by accident. I was in college, studying exercise science and personal training: I hated it. Two friends of mine, who had just graduated from the police academy said, "You're in shape. Why not join us?"

So, I did. (Yes, it was really that easy)

In June of 2007, I took the physical test. Back then, you actually had to be in shape to join the police force! I blew past all the tests because I was bodybuilding. Next thing I knew, I was in the police academy. I spent twelve years in that career. It wasn't my ultimate dream, but it gave me the money to pursue bodybuilding on the side, and I wanted to *protect and serve* my community.

This career choice would lead me to the greatest crisis of my life, where eight years straight of working the midnight shift crashed my hormone levels, upped my fat levels, and sent me spiraling into a depression I almost didn't come out of. It was this crisis that revealed to me the problem at the very heart of our medical industry:

Doctors today are too focused on symptom treatment and not symptom prevention.

I know this because when I went in to see my doctor, he prescribed me anti-depressants, of which one of the side-effects was *suicide*. What the hell? I'm feeling depressed, and you're treating me with symptom-masking, suicide-causing drugs?

My doctor wanted to layer on medication after medication. The train of medications would have gone something like this:

"Oh, you're feeling down? Here's an antidepressant."

"Your cholesterol's up? Here's a statin."

"Oh, your blood pressure's climbing? Here's something for that too."

And before long, I'd be juggling half a dozen prescriptions — each one treating the side effects of the last. What my doctor never said was:

"Let's look at your hormones," or

"Let's look at your diet." or

"Let's optimize your lifestyle before we drug you."

I knew that I needed more testosterone, but no regular doctor would prescribe me TRT because mine wasn't "low enough" according to FDA standards. I had a baseline test done when I was 19, so I knew I had dropped by over 50% since then. I reached out to a friend in the bodybuilding world who was running a rejuvenation clinic. I became a patient and got on TRT. Just like that, it changed everything.

I felt better. I was better. =

I was me again.

When I left law enforcement in 2018, I went to work at that clinic and helped build it into a powerhouse. That's how Aspire

Rejuvenation LLC eventually came to be. I was a patient before I ever became an owner.

I haven't looked back since.

THE FLU TRUTH

Ask anyone who's ever had the flu, "What do you want more than anything else in the world right now?"

"To not have the flu!"

It doesn't matter if you're a millionaire. If you're sick, getting well again matters more to you than money. After all, you can't enjoy your money or your success if you don't have your health. Health comes first; it's the difference between surviving and thriving.

Imagine health as the road you need to drive on to reach success, however you define success. Success to me is *fulfillment*, fulfillment of my purpose and God-given path. I want to accomplish what I've been born on this earth to accomplish.

What does success mean to you?

Are you on the road to that success,
or have you fallen from the path?

Maybe you've neglected your health, and your road is bumpy and full of potholes. Maybe you've fallen into the ditch, and you don't think you'll ever get back on your journey again. Maybe you're young and you're feeling good, and you want to ensure that you stay healthy and optimized all the way into your old age.

Wherever you are on the road of health, I am going to meet you where you're at to help you optimize your journey. This starts by changing your mindset about what health means.

Often, people will sacrifice their health to get more money, then they use that extra money to regain their health. This is crazy! Frankly, it's stupid. The truth is that you must optimize both at the same time to acquire both: **Health and wealth are inseparable expressions of success**.

They are also different things in this essential sense: Wealth is a perspective. Health is not. **Health is objective.** It's how your body functions, how you feel, how you perform, and how you look. You know when you're healthy. You know when you're not. Wealth can only derive from health, and not the other way around. Therefore, health must be our number one priority.

This book will take you from problem to solution, showing you how to uncover the root causes of illness, think critically in the doctor's office, and transform better health into a richer, fuller life.

WHAT THIS BOOK WILL DO FOR YOU

Every person's health journey is unique. Even identical twins can have drastically different hormone profiles based on their environment. We're all unique snowflakes (regardless of what "Fight Club" says). Seriously, if you don't realize that your health is unique to you, you'll just become a worn-down cog in a broken machine.

This is why my advice is always: **trust but verify**. Don't just blindly trust doctors. Don't just blindly trust me! This book will empower you with information, but it will also teach you how to think critically and choose for yourself. You'll learn how to recognize and reverse symptoms, take control of illness prevention, and design a lifestyle that restores lasting vitality. From there, we'll explore how true health becomes the foundation for wealth, influence, and a legacy that endures through your work, family, and future. Lastly, we'll ask the question – what do we optimize our lives for?

Here's a hint: it's not for our own sakes. Rather, we optimize our lives for the benefit of those around us. I'm forty years old as I write this. I want to still be able to run on the beach with my daughter when I'm forty-five, sixty-five, and eighty-five. For me, that is success. That is wealth. "Health is wealth" isn't just a saying, it's the hard truth.

The mission of *Operation Optimal* is to give you the achievable and actionable plan for your own success.

WHAT TO EXPECT IN THE CHAPTERS AHEAD

We're going to walk through a new approach to living. Your body talks to you. You'll learn how to listen, not just when it's screaming through illness or breakdowns, but when it's whispering, its subtlest signals. You'll discover how your hormones work, how they decline, and how you can restore them without relying on broken protocols or outdated science. We'll break down lifestyle fundamentals like diet, sleep, energy, discipline, aging, parenting, and sexual performance, while returning again and again to the one thing no pill can give you: *ownership of your health.*

You'll also hear my story. Not as a hero's tale, but as proof of what happens when you treat your body well, and what happens when you don't. Each season of my life taught me something about stress, decline, and recovery. That journey is a map, and I'm sharing it so you can navigate your own.

By the time we're done, you'll have the tools. You'll have the clarity. Most importantly, you'll have the mindset that nothing – not your doctor, not your schedule, not even your genetics – matters more than your decision to take control.

Here's a preview of each chapter ahead:

CHAPTER 2: GROWTH SIGNALS
Learn to decode the body's signals, distinguish between pain and growth, and build the awareness that transforms discomfort into strength.

CHAPTER 3: HACKING YOUR WAY TO HEALTH
Learn to reject shortcuts, lean into the productive hurt, and build a disciplined, whole-body routine that turns consistent training, clean nutrition, sleep discipline, and focused mornings into sustainable strength.

CHAPTER 4: THE TOLL OF STRESS

Learn what stress really is, how excess cortisol quietly wrecks your hormones and energy, and how to spot your personal signals early so you can convert negative stress into purposeful action with sleep, training, and better choices that restore balance, resilience, and control.

CHAPTER 5: BECOME YOUR BODY'S BEST EXPERT

Learn to walk into the exam room as your own expert, armed with the labs that matter, the questions that challenge assumptions, and a clear understanding of hormones, thyroid, and inflammation, so you shift from passive patient to informed owner of your health.

CHAPTER 6: KNOWING YOUR OPTIMAL & HOW TO GET THERE

Learn to define your personal optimal instead of settling for "normal," then reach it with targeted labs, slow-and-safe titration, lifestyle-first changes, and a reputable clinic so your hormones, energy, and mindset align.

CHAPTER 7: LONGEVITY & THE NEXT GENERATION

Learn what Blue Zones get right about long life and apply it with clean food and water, daily movement, less toxin and stress exposure, and firm parent-led modeling that protects kids' hormones and minds from junk inputs like processed food and screens.

CHAPTER 8: THE FUTURE OF MEDICINE

Discover how prevention-first, hormone-based, and regen-era-tive therapies, powered by new tech like biomarker tracking, gene-guided dosing, and AI, are replacing symptom-chasing with fast, personalized care.

CHAPTER 9: GUEST CHAPTER FROM DR. JOSEPH CLARK

Gain insight from Dr. Joseph Clark as he shares his expertise on hormones, prevention, and the future of truly patient-centered medicine.

CHAPTER 10: TURNING HEALTH INTO WEALTH

Learn how optimal health becomes the foundation for wealth, performance, and legacy by giving you the energy, focus, and presence to excel in business, relationships, and life itself.

CHAPTER 11: TURNING WEALTH INTO LASTING HAPPINESS

Learn to turn success into durable joy by pairing optimal health with Stoic self-mastery, intentional self-talk, daily gratitude, and authentic living that aligns your actions with purpose.

CHAPTER 12: LEGACY

Learn to turn your life into lasting impact by mentoring others, practicing daily consistency, aligning your actions with faith and honor, and taking radical ownership so your health, work, and values outlive you.

While this book has a clear progression from start to finish, you can read it in any order you like. Think of it as my personal mentorship to you. I'm not a medical doctor, but I am someone who's walked the path and knows what works. I trans-formed my own life for the best, and I want the best for you.

Read on, and **read in good health.**

CHAPTER 2

Growth Signals

Your body has a language all its own, and it speaks to you all the time. This is obvious when you really think about it:

- How did you know the stove was hot when you were a kid? You touched it: Ouch! That's your body speaking to you, "This hurts me."

- How did you know you love ice cream? You tasted it: Yum! That's your body speaking to you, "I like this."

- How did you know you ate too much ice cream? Ugh! You feel sick and sluggish! That's your body speaking to you, "Hey, treat me better!"

Here's what this looks like, with five more helpful examples:

LEARNING THE BODY'S SIGNALS

1. BODY SIGNAL

What your Body is Saying: *"Your weight, sleep quality, or airway may be compromised. I'm not getting the oxygen or recovery I need."*

Action Step 🏃 : Consider a sleep study, check for sleep apnea, and improve evening habits like reducing alcohol and late eating.

---

2. BODY SIGNAL

You climb a flight of stairs and feel chest tightness, shortness of breath, or unusual fatigue.

What your Body is Saying: *"Your heart is under strain. I can't keep up with demand."*

ACTION STEP 🏃 : Seek medical evaluation immediately. Prioritize heart health with testing, nutrition, and consistent cardio training.

---

3. BODY SIGNAL

You notice swollen ankles or frequent bloating after meals.

What your Body is Saying: *"Fluid is building up, or digestion isn't functioning properly. Something is off with circulation, kidneys, or your diet."*

ACTION STEP 🏃 : Monitor salt intake, increase hydration, and consult a doctor to rule out heart, kidney, or gut issues.

4. BODY SIGNAL

You often crave sugar and crash afterward, leaving you irritable and sluggish.

What your Body is Saying: *"My blood sugar is on a rollercoaster. I'm warning you about insulin resistance."*

Action Step 🏃 : Stabilize meals with protein, healthy fats, and fiber. Get fasting labs to check blood sugar and insulin levels.

---

5. BODY SIGNAL

You have frequent headaches, brain fog, and poor concentration.

What your Body is Saying: *"I'm inflamed, dehydrated, or missing key nutrients. Something is disrupting my balance."*

Action Step 🏃 : Track hydration, cut processed foods, and test for vitamin deficiencies or hormonal imbalances.

I first realized that my body was speaking to me during my puberty stage. When I went through puberty, I had a massive growth spurt. I remember being in a tremendous amount of pain from it, and from the hormonal fluctuations. My hormones were at an extremely high level, likely from genetics, but also from my diet.

We ate only Mediterranean and homemade foods. My mom was cooking everything, so we weren't going out and eating anything processed. In the U.S., fast food was all around us, but we couldn't afford it! That's right, we grew up so poor that it was cheaper to eat healthy. *McDonald's* was a luxury when I was growing up.

Going through puberty, this is what I was hearing from my body: My energy levels were through the roof. My joint pain was through the roof. I had a really high sex drive. Teenagers are often angry, and I definitely had anger spurts too. Here's the thing, these physical and mental *symptoms* were *signals* from my body, all telling me one thing:

"Start working out."

So, I did. I started working out when I was 13. I didn't know it at the time, but I was listening to my body's language. **Your body is your most valuable and intimate mentor**. If you listen and follow it, it will never lead you astray.

LEARNING THE GYM LIFE

At the gym, I was taken under the wing of several mentors. They taught me about what to eat, how to build muscle, and how to be healthy. This was before all the current research and studies came out saying that *the more muscle you have, the longer you're going to live*. Dr. Gabrielle Lyon calls muscle, **the organ of longevity**, and she's right. Her data-driven work shows that muscle mass is the best predictor of longevity.[1]

---

[1] Gabrielle Lyon, Forever Strong: A New, Science-Based Strategy for Aging Well (New York: Simon & Schuster/Atria Books, October 17, 2023), 400.

This explains how guys like Jack LaLanne were working out until the day they died at the age of 91. You don't think he was on HRT? Of course he was!

THE VALUE OF COMPETITION: PAIN VS. HURT

Youth is the massive life hack that nobody takes advantage of. Before 25, your hormones are at peak performance, and if you're eating right and training, you thrive. I realized that weightlifting was about way more than solving pain. It was about more than looking good for girls. It was about *competition*. Everyone needs competition in their lives, some more than others. Competition elevates all of us.

An important figure in my life at the gym, the man who kept me competitive and even made me train legs 2-3 times a week (because I told him I hated it!) was Don Divito.

Don mentored me from the time I was about 13 until I was 17. He used to say, "Are you in pain, or does it just hurt?" If it hurt, he'd say, "Good. Push through it."

Don taught me that there's a big difference between **pain** and **hurt**.

This is another way that your body talks to you. Pain is your body telling you to stop. Pain will point to things like injury, illness, and bad techniques. Are you in pain? Stop doing that thing. In contrast, *hurt* is your body telling you that you're growing. Are you working out properly, and it's hurting? Good! All good things hurt at first: success, starting a business, starting a diet, the hurt you go through with these things is just the price you pay for the growth.

Don was tough. Out of the goodness of his heart, he taught us everything from discipline to posture. If he saw us slouching in the gym, he'd say something crazy like, "I'll strap a bungee cord from your neck to your asshole," and we believed he'd do it! It wasn't that we were afraid of him; we respected him. We didn't want to disappoint him.

Don had type-1 diabetes, which is genetic, not lifestyle-based. The doctors told him that he'd be dead by 50. He said, "No," to that and kept right on training and living his healthy kick-ass lifestyle. He lived into his 70s and was in great shape the whole way through. He was happy and fulfilled. Don trusted what his body told him, not what his doctors demanded. Don was even repping a high-protein diet, active lifestyle, and biomechanics long before most people were even thinking that way. He was decades ahead of his time.

Don't ever use a diagnosis, illness, or anxiety – no matter how harsh and depressing it is – as an excuse to live unhealthily. We live our lives to the fullest, and we do that through empowering ourselves for health.

From **discipline** to **posture**, live your life like Don!

PAIN IS A SIGNAL, NOT A SYMPTOM

Pain isn't the problem. It's the message. Most people silence it instead of asking what it's trying to say. That's why I don't call it the medical industry. It's the pain industry, built to manage pain, not to heal it!

Most doctors made pain a central symptom and then made it their job to erase it. In reality, pain is a signal. It's not something to medicate away every time. If something hurts because it's healing, you have to push through that. If some-thing hurts because you're growing, grow!

But doctors tell you not to move, but to "Rest, rest, rest."

That kills people. A body only ever at rest is a dead one. A body in motion stays in motion. We were meant to move. Muscles are the biggest organ in the body. If you stop using them, everything suffers. Rest isn't always the answer.

Doctors will often treat the symptoms instead of asking what's causing it. They won't ask about your food. They won't ask about your genetics. Why are you on blood pressure meds if you've never had a test for MTHFR mutation (a gene that affects how the body processes vitamin B9)?[2,3]

Did you know that high blood pressure can often be corrected with the right combination of vitamins? Most people never hear that from their doctor because the system isn't built to focus on prevention or root causes. It's built to prescribe.

Take Dr. Clark Store, for example. He battled high blood pressure for fifty years. One day, instead of relying on more

---

2   American College of Medical Genetics and Genomics, "Lack of Evidence for MTHFR Polymorphism Testing," Genetics in Medicine 15, no. 2 (2013): 153-56, recommending against routine clinical MTHFR testing.

3   Maun, A. "Treating the Cause, Not the Symptoms." Journal of Clinical & Translational Endocrinology (2023). On the risk of medical practice focusing on symptom suppression rather than root causes.

medication, he tried a methylated vitamin protocol that targeted the body's natural chemistry. Within months, his blood pressure normalized, and he was off cholesterol meds for good. So why don't more doctors talk about that?

Because there's no profit in a solution that ends the prescription cycle?[4]

Well, some doctors have been brainwashed too. They're not malicious, just misled. Doctors are trained to treat symptoms, not prevent disease. They do what they're trained to do.

We have to stop thinking of pain as something evil. Sometimes pain is the only way your body knows how to talk to you. The difference is whether you're dealing with harm or adaptation. If it's pain — stop. If it just hurts — lean in.

That's where **growth** is.

LISTEN TO YOUR BODY AND HEAL

If you've been ignoring your body's signals, or if you've been desensitized to your pain and depression, the first step is to *start moving*. Return to what you did as a kid. Play outside. Get your shoes on and shoot a basketball. Go swing on the swings. If you grew up video-gaming, think about what you loved in games. Wasn't your character leveling up and getting

---

4 S.D. Amenyah et al., "DNA Methylation of Hypertension-Related Genes and Effect of Riboflavin Supplementation in Adults with the MTHFR 677TT Genotype," *Journal of Hypertension & Related Research* (2021).

stronger in the game? Great! Now apply that to real life. Level up your real body. Stop drinking soda. Cut the chips. Take one baby step at a time. Stop snoozing your alarm. Drink more water. Take back control.

As soon as you see results, your confidence builds. Then you start asking the right questions. Why should I take this medication? Instead, why don't I try a lifestyle solution? That curiosity brings freedom.

That's health **ownership**.

THIS APPLIES TO YOUR MENTAL HEALTH TOO

You want to talk about the real mental health revolution?

It starts in your bloodstream. **Fix your hormones.**

Hormones are another way that our body talks to us. Often, people ignore this until the conversation of the body turns into something like a shouting match. I'm talking about what breaks most people, both men and women: menopause and andropause.

Did you know that postmenopausal women have the highest rates of osteoporosis, dementia, and depression out of anyone?[5]

---

[5] Délio M. Conde et al., "Menopause and Cognitive Impairment: A Narrative Review of Current Knowledge," World Journal of Clinical Cases 9, no. 22 (2021): 6297–6311, https://www. ncbi.nlm.nih.gov/pmc/articles/PMC8394691/.

It's not a mystery; it's hormone collapse. Put meno-pausal women on bioidentical hormones and watch what happens. They feel 25 again. They sleep. They smile. They think clearly. No more SSRIs (a class of antidepressant medications commonly prescribed for depression and anxiety disorders). No more guesswork.

It's the same with men. Actually, most men have never even heard the term **andropause** before. Most know it as a midlife crisis. And men buy themselves a new corvette or leave their wives of thirty years. What are they doing? Besides being stupid, they're seeking something that they don't understand.

It's not just that they've lost an attraction for their wives. It's that they have attraction to nothing. It isn't psycho-logical, it's hormonal. It's testosterone crashing. What do doctors give men when this happens?

Viagra. Or Cialis.

Those pills are a *multi-trillion-dollar industry*. And it was all based on heart medication. They're vasodilators. Those drugs vasodilate the whole body, not just the penis. It doesn't actually fix the problem; it just treats the symptoms. What would fix the problem?

Testosterone.

Why don't doctors prescribe testosterone? Because they're not taught to. Because Big Pharma can't patent testosterone. Big Pharma isn't interested unless it turns a profit, and the mental health industry is one of the most profitable industries on earth.[67]

HORMONAL STRENGTH IS MENTAL STRENGTH

I've seen VA patients come into my clinic carrying grocery bags literally full of pills. Pills for depression, anxiety, PTSD, you name it. They usually have sharply declining testos-terone levels. Within months of optimizing their hormones, they're off all meds. They cry for joy. They feel alive again. And then they're angry:

"Why didn't anyone check this!? Why didn't they even ask me about this? Why didn't they even put it in the blood test?"

The system isn't built to *fix* pain. Not even for our vet-erans! The system is built to *manage* pain. Big Medicine has been bought and sold by Big Pharma, and Big Pharma says that for depression, you take depression medication. Of course, there are real people with real mental health prob-lems that require pills, like schizophrenia. I have nothing against that. But at the same time, I can tell you that the men-tal health industry would shrink overnight if doctors stopped looking for *symptoms* and started looking for *signals* that point to a root cause.

We have to teach people something different. How you felt at eighteen should be how you feel today. Don't accept decline as

---

[6] See *Pharmaceutical Innovations* and in W. Grimes, "Perverse Results from Pharma-ceutical Patents," showing how patent strategy skews R&D priorities.

[7] See G.K. Jasuja et al., "Understanding the Context of High- and Low-Testosterone Use: System and Clinician Factors in Veterans Health Administration," *Journal of Clinical Endocrinology & Metabolism* (2019).

normal. It's not. You can turn the clock back. You can heal. You can feel amazing again, not "good for your age," but *good*. Period.

It's the same thing with mental health as with your bodily health. Pain is signals, not symptoms. And just as you can listen to your body, you can listen to your mind.

LISTENING TO YOUR MIND: STOICISM

Stoicism is a philosophy and a way of life which teaches us how to know ourselves. It's not about suppressing our feelings. Rather, it's about taking radical ownership of our thoughts and actions, allowing us to feel fully and then to act accordingly.

Dan Sullivan, one of the world's foremost experts on entrepreneurship in action, says that preserving your confi-dence is key to your mental health. You do that through self-talk. How you talk to yourself is how you master your mind.

Everyone has that inner voice. Most people's inner voice is brutal and mean. But you are that voice! So, you can change the narrative of yourself. Stoicism helped me with that. It's not about suppressing emotion; it's about mastering it. Feel it, understand it, but don't let it control you. That's power. My mom taught me this before I had a name for it.

"Tomo, you can't control the world around you without first controlling yourself," she told me.

I guess my mom must have read the Roman Emperor, Marcus Aurelius:

"You have power over your mind, not outside events. Realize this, and you will find strength." (Meditations 6.48)

If you're sad and can't do anything about it, *move on.* If you can do something, do it. Don't sit and wallow in your emotions. Acknowledge the feeling, then take action. A mind in motion stays in motion.

Many people today seem to be in a place where feeling like the victim is the place to be. They hear things like, "You're not fat, you're not obese. It's just genetics. It's just your external circumstances."

F#ck off! If you're obese, you're obese. It's a disease. Let's help you get well.

If we're talking about mental health, the excuse we often hear and use for ourselves is *depression.* I know what this is like, I've been *depressed* before. Here's the thing: it wasn't real, not in the sense of an incurable disease that needed pills to treat. What I didn't know was that my testosterone levels were one third the level they should have been. I optimized my hormones and boom! No more depression.[8]

Depression is a signal pointing to your situation. I was going through a divorce at the time; I was *sad.* That's okay. It's normal and healthy to experience the emotion of sadness. Just go through it. Don't repress it until it becomes depres-

---

8 For a study backing my claim here, see Walther, Andreas, et al. "Association of Testosterone Treatment With Alleviation of Depressive Symptoms in Men: A Systematic Review and Meta-analysis of 27 Randomized Controlled Trials." *JAMA Psychiatry* (2019).

sion. Remember what Don said: **Push through the hurt to get to the healthy.**

Jim Rohn, a renowned public speaker, put it this way:

"Don't wish it was easier.
Wish you were better.

Don't wish for less problems.
Wish for more skills.

Don't wish for less challenge.
Wish for more wisdom."

ACTION STEPS

Your mindset changes your mind, and your mind changes your world. Here's three action steps you can take today towards optimizing your physical and mental health:

1. MOVE YOUR BODY EVERY DAY

Walk, stretch, lift, or play. Revisit move-ments you enjoyed as a kid (shoot hoops, go for a jog, swing at the park). Start simple and be consistent.

2. DIFFERENTIATE BETWEEN PAIN AND HURT

When discomfort shows up, pause and ask: Is this pain (harm) or hurt (growth)? If it hurts, lean in. If it's pain, investigate the root cause and adapt.

3. MASTER YOUR SELF-TALK

Monitor your internal dialogue. Speak to yourself with clarity and control.

Practice this Stoic reflection: What can I control? What must I accept?

CHAPTER 3

Hacking Your Way to Health

The road to optimal health isn't a sprint. There are no shortcuts or hacks. It's a marathon. Every step counts. This chapter is about avoiding shortcuts, leaning into the hurt, and bringing your whole body and mind to bear in your daily routine. We'll get into workout tips, diet, and motivation. Don't wait around.

Let's get **moving**.

BRING YOUR WHOLE BODY TO YOUR ROUTINE

The body is capable of incredible things if treated right. When you're in the gym, you can see those incredible things happen tangibly and immediately. This is stating the obvious: You work on your arms, they get bigger. It's the same with your chest and anything else. But many people will focus on just one area of their body and neglect the rest. This is a mistake!

You have to work **your entire body**
to get the best body possible.

I'm tall and I have long legs, so I had to work out my leg muscles two-three times a week, and it sucked! We all dread leg-day. I really hated the way my calves looked, so I made a training protocol. I gave myself the hardest challenge possible: I would do psychotically-heavy calf raises and calf presses. Then I would take a day off and then do another leg day of super high volume. Rinse and repeat. I never missed a day, and one year later, I had the calves I wanted to have.

Lean into the hurt to get to the health.

Here's the takeaway: never train just one part of your body. You want bigger arms? Train your legs three days a week, your arms for two, and your chest for two. Look at a professional sprinter as an example. They have built legs, a sculpted chest, and are strong everywhere. They don't isolate; they integrate. Training the whole body conditions every part to perform better.

Your legs are your largest muscle group, the second largest is your back, while your arms and chest are your smallest. So why put 100% effort into the smallest muscle group of your body? People skip the hard and avoid the hurt. People want shortcuts.

There are no shortcuts to health.

There are no shortcuts to wealth.

There are no shortcuts to legacy.

THE SHORTCUT WE ALL THINK OF: STEROIDS.

I want to be clear: I do not recommend steroids for personal use. It's one thing if you're Lebron James, or another top athlete that wouldn't survive playing at the level they do without some form of anabolic, under the guidance of top trainers, dieticians, and doctors. For the rest of us, steroids are a dangerous and often tempting shortcut to gains.

Using steroids means taking synthetic anabolic compounds, usually in unsafe doses, to blow past the body's natural limits and force muscle growth. Using HRT means restoring your body to healthy, optimal hormone levels that already exist in your physiology. Steroids are about artificial enhancement. HRT is about natural replacement. One breaks you down over time. The other builds you back to where you're supposed to be.

When I was coming up in the bodybuilding world, I wanted shortcuts more than anybody. I wanted the steroids and all the growth hormones I could get my hands on. Luckily, I held off until I truly needed it, when the signs of declining testosterone started showing:

- Low energy no matter how much I rested

- Harder time building and keeping muscle

- Sluggish recovery after workouts

- Mood swings and irritability

- Drop-off in my motivation, both in the gym and in life

The first time I took it was a rush. I knew what everyone had been talking about. I'm not going to lie and pretend I never went overboard. I did. And when I did, I learned. Every failure, to me, is just a lesson. I thought I could out-train and out-diet a higher dose. I was wrong. Instead of looking better, I ended up looking worse.

I took more HRT-based doses: testosterone, growth hormones, and prescription oxandrolone. In earlier cycles, I was even running things like trenbolone. The truth? I felt like shit, and I looked worse and worse. My training intensity dropped. The shortcuts weren't pushing me harder; they were dragging me down with the mindset: "I'm on the shortcut, so I don't need to push myself."

For context, oxandrolone is better known as Anavar. Guys chase it because it's supposed to give lean, "dry" muscle gains with less water retention. In reality, without discipline in the gym and kitchen, it does very little. I learned that the hard way. There was a tangible price to pay. A lot of people in the bodybuilding industry will overdose and start to have detrimental effects like:

- High cholesterol

- High blood pressure

- Night sweats and other sleeping problems

- Depression

I don't understand the idea that any of these symptoms is worth it just *for muscles.* Fortunately, I never overdosed enough to get these symptoms. When I cut my dosages, and got on more minimal stuff, that's when I dialed in with cardio, better food, and all the other things I hadn't dialed in on before but should have. I dialed in because I had to. There were no shortcuts to fall back on as excuses.

I was no Ronnie Coleman, but I sure as hell was Tomo Marjanovic, the best me I could be!

HORMONE THERAPY ISN'T A SHORTCUT

We compare ourselves to other people, and that's what often prompts us to take shortcuts. We want to (immediately) be that other person who's way ahead of us in some way.

It's a common misconception that Hormone Optimization Therapy is another shortcut like steroids, Ozempic, and other weight loss drugs. HRT is not just something you put in your body and forget about. You still have to put in your whole body and whole mind effort into your health journey. This is why I want HRT to be accessible to everyone, and that's why I'm writing this book! Whether it's weight loss drugs, steroids, or even my own HRT clinic, people are looking for shortcuts. I hate it when young guys come into my clinic and say things like, 'I want to take testosterone! I just want to get a little boost on my bicep here. :)'

This drives me nuts!

If you're 25, chances are your deficiencies are in your lifestyle, not your hormones. There are exceptions, such as a genetic issue, or something physically wrong with your HPTA (hypothalamic pituitary axis). But usually, it's lifestyle. So, I don't want to see you in my clinic! Improving your lifestyle improves your hormones. Get into the gym. Put in more than 15% effort. Don't spend your time texting or surfing TikTok. HRT isn't going to get you 'gains', working out like a beast will.

As an example, HRT is for the dad that goes out every single day to do roofing. That dude is breaking his back, on back-to-back work every single day to support his family. Maybe he's in his late 40s and he can't roof as quick as he used to. Maybe his sex drive is falling. Maybe he's feeling depressed. Is it *cheating* for him to be on HRT and feel younger and stronger? Is it a *shortcut* that he can use growth hormones to repair his broken body, and do a stem cell treatment once a year? No way! I want that HRT for him because he wants, and deserves, to live his life to the fullest again.

HRT is not steroids. It's not a shortcut. But it seems like it is to some people, because we don't know to recognize the difference between a health shortcut and a health *tool*. The best of the best know how to use these tools *as tools* to train.

LOOKING UP TO THE BEST OF THE BEST OF THE BEST

It doesn't matter how many steroids you take. It doesn't matter how many shortcuts you take. You're never going to look like Arnold Schwarzenegger. You're never going to look like Ronnie Coleman or Lee Haney. These guys were genetic phenotypes, and guess what? They trained like f#cking animals (that's my one curse word for this chapter)! These guys were perfection personified in the realm of bodybuilding. Of course there was steroid use involved. They were at that level where they would have been almost as fantastic without them. But steroids weren't their secret. What was?

They had the courage
to be their best selves.

It's the same thing with other sports. Professional athletes are using things, including MLB, NBA, NFL or NHL. They are all using something, whether it's stem cells, HRT, peptides, all three, or things that we don't even know about yet. However, just because they (allegedly) use these things, doesn't mean we should. We train for the level we want to reach *as the people we are*. Don't train to be Lebron James, and don't desire *to be* Lebron.

Train to be you.
Desire to be your best you.

All that being said, it's good to look to your favorite athlete as inspiration, even as a kind of mentor. For me, that's the great Ronnie Coleman, who won the Mr. Olympia title a record-tying eight times, from 1998 to 2005. That guy never skipped the gym. That guy never gave less than 150 percent effort. He squatted 800 pounds for two reps, never skipped cardio, and never missed a meal.[9]

"Yeah buddy!" he'd say; that became his trademark. He was bodybuilding perfection. Yeah, he was on serious anabolic, but it wasn't about cutting corners. He took it to be the best of the best of the best. And he destroyed and broke his body nearly to the point of crippling it in the process. When people ask him, 'Do you regret it?'

Here's what Ronnie Coleman said:

"I didn't go heavy enough. One time I was squatting 800. I thought it'd be heavy, but after the first rep I'm like, is this 800? Did another, still easy. But I had it in my mind to do 2, and afterward I'm like, man, I could've done 3 or 4 more. That still bothers me."[10]

That quote blows me away. After all the pain, after a lifetime of bodybuilding and surgeries, Ronnie's one regret is that he didn't squat enough? Those same squats destroyed his back, and he still thinks he had one more in him?

This is exactly what I'm talking about when I say you shouldn't want to be your favorite top athletes (unless you are one), but you can take inspiration from them. Ronnie Coleman is insane! But I love the dedication, and I try and model my life around that kind of grit.

---

[9] "Ronnie Coleman's Heaviest Lifts Ever," BarBend, accessed September 2025, https://barbend.com/ronnie-coleman-heaviest-lifts-ever

[10] Coleman, Ronnie. 2022. Ronnie Coleman on His Only Regret: Not Doing More Reps with 800 Pounds. Interview by Muscle Mind Media. TikTok video, 1:00. April 13, 2022.

HOW TO RECOGNIZE HEALTH TOOLS *AS TOOLS*

Is doing an ice bath cheating? Is taking a cold shower cheating? Where do we draw the line between health *hacks* and *hacking* our way to health?

My rule of thumb is:

✓   **It's available**

✓   **It's safe**

✓   **It's motivating you to do more
(not giving you excuses)**

✓   **It's challenging you**

If your health hack checks these four boxes, it's not a hack – it's a tool, and it's one that you should use. We can apply this rule of thumb to a controversial topic in the health world today: peptides.

Peptides are naturally occurring amino acid chains that are already present in your body. BPC 157, for example, is a synthetic peptide derived from a protein found in human gastric juice. It was invented by a Croatian (go Croatia!) and has been around since the 80s. This peptide is also known as The Wolverine because it can heal soft tissue damage rapidly.[11] We've used it very successfully in my clinic. Is it cheating to use this tool if you need it?

[11] M. Józwiak et al., "Multifunctionality and Possible Medical Application of the Stable Gastric Peptide BPC 157 (Molecular Basis)," *Pharmaceuticals* 18, no. 2 (2025): 185, https://doi.org/10.3390/ph18020185

Use the table above to answer that question for yourself.

Here's the crazy thing: it's hard to find a single bad side effect. And that's not me sugarcoating it. The reason is simple, your body already knows what to do with peptides. They're chains of amino acids, the same building blocks you're made of. Unlike synthetic drugs that hijack your system, peptides usually work by amplifying what your body is designed to do in the first place. That's why, when you look through the research, the "risks" section is almost blank. It doesn't mean you can be reckless, but it explains why so many people call BPC 157 one of the safest performance and recovery tools out there.

Whatever health tool you use, it's how you use it that matters. Safety first. Did you know that you can overdose on aspirin? 10x the safe dosage and your liver shuts down. Then you die. The point I'm trying to make here is that it's your mindset that matters. Taking the same drugs with different mindsets applied produces dramatically different outcomes.

Any hormone, peptide, or even steroid you take should be considered well, consulted with a healthcare professional, and always applied with the mindset that *this is a tool, not a shortcut*. Your body is a perfect and beautiful machine, and you want to use this perfect beautiful machine in the best way possible. We need to optimize our health now before it's too late. Increase your lifespan before your lifespan gets cut short due to your poor lifestyle. We are already seeing the societal cost of this.

Testosterone levels in men are getting lower and lower with every generation.[12] Our grandfathers and our great grandfathers had two to three times higher testosterone than we do today. For example, I had almost 1500ng/dL when I was measured. My great-grandfather surely had a much higher number! Maybe even 4500 ng/dL. He must have been the Croatian Ronnie Coleman!

In all seriousness, you have to take the best possible advantage of the tools you have. You have to have the mindset to see them as tools, not shortcuts. Lastly, you have to put in the work. I'll say it again, lean into the hurt to get to the healthy. This next part of the chapter is going to give you specifics on how to do just that.

DIETARY

Make sure that what you're intaking is clean. Clean is healthy. Eat, drink, and consume with purpose. Your purpose should be to *eat to be healthy*. This also goes for what you feed your mind. Endless Tik-Tok scrolling is just processed food for the brain.

Next, be informed. Do things like gut health tests, food sensitivity, blood vitamin and mineral tests. Find out what your body is missing and what your body has intolerance for. Whatever your specifics are, you'll likely need to be eating omnivorously. Humans are not carnivores or vegans (sorry!). These

---

12 Thomas G. Travison et al., "A Population-Level Decline in Serum Testosterone Levels in American Men," Journal of Clinical Endocrinology & Metabolism 92, no. 1 (2007): 196–202, https://doi.org/10.1210/jc.2006-1375.

dietary extremes are not the right way to be healthy and maintain healthiness, although they can serve as corrective diets for small amounts of time.

Our stomachs can't even digest half of the vegetables that we eat.[13] Similarly, meat only does not provide all of our necessary nutrients.[14]

Follow the middle way between these two extremes.

I like to eat at least 5 pieces of fruit every day. In fact, as I'm writing this, I just had a Kiwi, some jackfruit, and a peach. I'm gonna go eat steak in a little bit too. I eat high protein with a supplement of natural sugars, usually from fruits. Whatever your specific diet is, stay away from processed foods and refined sugars if you want to live an optimal life.

EXERCISE

Everyone has a work schedule that's unique to them. But whatever your situation is, you must make time for exercise. Saying 'I just don't have time to work out' is unacceptable. If you're on a normal 9-5ish schedule, go to sleep earlier to wake up earlier, and get your fitness/health routine done. The morning is always the best time for anything. The morning is when you are fresh, not distracted by the world, life, technology, family, or whatever your distractions are.

---

[13] Hans Konrad Biesalski, "Digestibility Issues of Vegetable versus Animal Proteins: Protein and Amino Acid Requirements—Functional Aspects," *Food and Nutrition Bulletin* 32, no. 3 (2011): 150–154.

[14] Miki Ben-Dor et al., "Assessing the Nutrient Composition of a Carnivore Diet," *Nutrients* 16, no. 13 (2024): 1857.

Your exercise routine doesn't have to be long, and it doesn't even have to be in a gym. Think about how many squats, push-ups, sit-ups, etc. you can do in 20 minutes. That's all it takes, and you don't even need any equipment. You just need proper sleep and the discipline to follow through.

SLEEP DISCIPLINE

Sleep is the most important thing for your body's recovery. Your circadian rhythm is also important as it relates to your hormones, how your body processes work, and how your brain works. Everything is better when you are sleeping properly. If you've ever suffered from insomnia, you know what I'm talking about.

Not including naps (which are great if you can get them), make sure you're sleeping 6 to 8 hours a day. This sounds simple, and you've probably heard this many times before. Yet still, most people sleep like they're lying on a bed of nails. They take sleeping pills just to get by. If this sounds like you, examine your lifestyle first and eliminate any causes of why you might be sleeping poorly such as:

- Too much screen time before bed

- Not getting exercise prior to sleep

- Poor diet (processed foods, artificial sugars)

- Not maintaining a regular circadian rhythm[15]

---

[15] Qianyun Zhong et al., "Electronic Screen Use and Sleep Duration and Timing in Adults," *JAMA Network Open* 8, no. 9 (September 2025): e2331993.

If you eliminate all of these things and you're still sleeping poorly, then get a sleep assessment to find out more information.

The prime time for people to make excuses or take shortcuts in life is
the first moment of the day.

We all know what this feels like. You're having a pleasant dream and then RING goes the alarm clock. So, you hit snooze. This is a big mistake because now your first action of your day is a compromise, an excuse to be lazy. Here's my foolproof advice for how to not do this:

Don't keep your alarm clock within arm's reach!

Keep your alarm, whether it's your phone or otherwise, within walking distance. This means that you have to take several steps away from your bed to turn it off. Well, maybe it's not completely foolproof. If you consciously go back to bed after *walking to turn off your alarm*, then you're just lazy. If this is happening, put your gym clothes on top of your alarm. Add as many steps as possible before you turn it off; do anything you can to motivate yourself to wake up at the time you set for yourself. That way, you can start every day with a victory.

Next, take a cold shower or get some cold water in your face right in the morning. ZAP! You're now right awake. It's a slap to the face.

Next, do some kind of physical activity. It could be as simple as twenty minutes of indoor exercise, walking the dog, to a full on gym workout. Whatever you have time and ability to do, do it. Start your day with purposeful movement of your body. Exercise energizes you; it doesn't make you tired. Whoever left the gym after a real workout feeling depressed, sluggish, and unmotivated?

Hell no! You leave the gym feeling like you can take on the world, and you can! An optimal morning gives you optimal health and perspective right from the get-go. The right morning routine sets your whole day up for success.

Don't let an excuse like, "I don't have time to work out" get in the way of that. It's just not true. Start by trimming the fat. The average person spends nearly seven hours a day on their smartphone, with constant pickups throughout the day.[16]

That's an enormous block of time that could be redirected into movement, training, or simply taking better care of yourself. In addition, most people wake up in the morning and they spend between 20 and 40 minutes on their phone or watching TV. They waste a tremendous amount of time on their cell phones and television in the morning. What does that add up to?

- About **3 hr. 20min per week**

- About **15 hours per month**

- About **7 days straight per year!**

---

[16] AHM Bradley et al., "Stress and Mood Associations With Smartphone Use in Young Adults," *PMC* (2023)

Reading these stats should be like a splash of cold water on your face. What if you used all that time for a quick workout instead. Optimizing your morning optimizes your health. So, get started tomorrow morning!

BUDGETING FOR HEALTH

There's a common misconception that eating healthy is more expensive than eating unhealthy. It's wrong. Eating healthy is the more affordable option. To prove this point, I'm going to offer you a side-by-side comparison between the average American's grocery receipt vs. one that's built around healthy and pure foods only. This is based on the latest data available from the time of writing this, July 2025.

GROCERY BASKET COST COMPARISON TABLE
(MID-2025 AVERAGE PRICES)

	Average American Basket (Processed-Food Heavy)	Healthy Whole-Food Basket (Minimally Processed)
Produce	Bananas (2 lb @ $0.66/lb) = $1.32; Potatoes (5 lb @ $0.98/lb) = $4.90. **Total ≈ $6.20**	Bananas (3 lb @ $0.66/lb) = $1.98; Apples (2 lb @ $1.20/lb) = $2.40; Carrots (2 lb @ $1.00/lb) = $2.00; Tomatoes (1 lb @ $1.79/lb) = $1.79; Oranges (2 lb @ $1.79/lb) = $3.58. **Total ≈ $11.80**
Protein	Ground beef, 80/20 (2 lb @ $6.25/lb) = $12.50; Hot dogs (1 lb) ≈ $3.50. **Total ≈ $16.00**	Chicken breast (2 lb @ $4.20/lb) = $8.40; Salmon fillet (2 lb @ ~$7.15/lb) ≈ $14.30; Black beans (1 lb) ≈ $2.00; Eggs (1 dozen) ≈ $3.60. **Total ≈ $28.30**
Grains	White bread (1 loaf) = $1.85; Sugary cereal (1 box) ≈ $4.00; Frozen pizza (1 pack) ≈ $6.00. **Total ≈ $11.85**	Whole wheat bread (1 loaf) = $2.70; Oatmeal (18 oz) ≈ $2.50; Brown rice (2 lb) ≈ $2.12. **Total ≈ $7.30**

Dairy	Whole milk (1 gal) ≈ $4.17; Processed cheese slices (1 lb) ≈ $4.90; Ice cream (½ gal) ≈ $6.40. **Total ≈ $15.47**	Low-fat milk (1 gal) ≈ $4.17; Greek yogurt, plain (32 oz) ≈ $4.00. **Total ≈ $8.17**
Snacks & Sweets	Potato chips (16 oz) = $6.80; Chocolate chip cookies (1 lb) = $5.26; Oreos (14 oz) ≈ $5.00; Candy bars (multi-pack) ≈ $6.00. **Total ≈ $23.06**	Almonds or mixed nuts (1 lb) ≈ $8.00; plus snacking from produce. **Total ≈ $8.00**
Beverages	Soda (2 × 2-liter bottles @ $1.75 each) = $3.50; Sports drinks (6-pack) ≈ $7.50; Sweetened iced tea jug ≈ $4.50. **Total ≈ $15.50**	Water (tap/filtered) = $0; Herbal tea ≈ $0. **Total $0**
Frozen/Prepared Meals	Chicken nuggets (32 oz bag) ≈ $8.50; TV dinner (2-pack) ≈ $7.50. **Total ≈ $16.00**	*Not included.*

TOTALS

- **Average American Basket (junk-heavy): ≈ $104.10**
- **Healthy Whole-Food Basket: ≈ $63.57**

KEY TAKEAWAY

- That's a **~39% difference** in cost.

- The junk-heavy cart blows past $100 largely due to snacks, sugary drinks, and frozen convenience meals.

- The healthy basket — built around produce, lean proteins, beans, grains, and yogurt — stays in the mid-$60s.

As you can see, most people are overspending on processed junk, fast food, and convenience meals without even realizing it. When you build your diet around clean, whole foods like rice, beans, eggs, produce, frozen veggies, you'll actually spend less per month than the average American. According to the latest numbers, **a healthy grocery list can cost around 40% less per trip than junk-food choices.** Don't let the lie keep you broke and sick.

Discipline at the grocery store saves money and your health. It can even improve your cholesterol, hormone levels, energy, and mental health.

BE HEALTHY... AND ENJOY LIFE!

The goal of all of this is not masochism, putting yourself through hurt for its own sake. No way! You go through the hurt to get to the healthy, and *you go through the healthy to get to the happy.* I'm a big proponent of enjoying your life. I went to Abu Dhabi recently, guess what I had for lunch when I was over there?

A Big Mac!

I just wanted one, and I knew they weren't as processed as they are in the USA. So, I chose to enjoy life, to have my Big Mac and eat it too. My point is that I'm not telling you that you have to live a super strict lifestyle like Bryan Johnson, who spends literally millions of dollars per year just to live longer. What I'm teaching here is: Make the right choices.

If you don't know what the right choices are, then seek out good information. Assess your intake. Measure your output. Ask questions like, what am I getting out of this? Is this working for me? Your body is already answering those questions for you. If you haven't read chapter 2 yet, take some time to. The takeaway from that chapter is: your body is your greatest source of wisdom and mentorship when it comes to your own health. Every action and every decision you make, whether it's what you eat, how you move, how late you stay up, or who you surround yourself with, either pushes you closer to your goal or pulls you further away from it. That is the lens you need to see through. Is this action getting me closer to the life I want, or is it keeping me stuck in the same patterns I am trying to escape? If you can get honest with yourself in that moment, the answer is usually obvious.

The takeaway from this chapter is: There's no hack to health; you have *to hack* your way to health with the determination, discipline, and positivity it would take to chop down the Amazon rainforest using only a handaxe. That's a powerful metaphor. Now imagine that you're also the trees, and for every one drop of effort you put in, you get twice as strong.

ACTION STEPS

Here's three action steps you can take today towards optimizing your physical and mental health:

1. **TRAIN YOUR WHOLE BODY, NOT JUST YOUR FAVORITES**

   Avoid muscle imbalances and half-effort routines. Don't skip leg day, back day, or cardio. A strong body is a balanced body, so commit to a weekly split that hits every major muscle group, and double down on the ones you usually avoid.

2. **ELIMINATE ONE SHORTCUT YOU'RE RELYING ON**

   Identify a habit that feels productive but is really avoidance, like pre-workout instead of real rest, gear instead of grit, or scrolling instead of sweating. Replace it with a tool that pushes you: cold showers, a disciplined routine, or simply pushing harder in your next workout.

3. **START YOUR MORNING WITH A WIN**

   Set your alarm out of reach and prep your gear the night before. When you wake up, move immediately, no phone, no delay. Try this: cold water to the face, 20 bodyweight reps, then a clean whole food meal. Start strong, and the rest of your day will follow.

CHAPTER 4

The Toll of Stress

I was a cop for twelve years. The stress of that profession took a toll on my body and mind that I wasn't informed enough yet to deal with. Knowing what I know now, the warning signs of stress (signals, my body talking to me) are super clear.

WHAT STRESS IS: CORTISOL

Cortisol is a steroid hormone, often called the stress hormone, produced by your adrenal glands. If you know what an adrenaline rush feels like, you know what cortisol feels like. It plays a vital role in regulating various bodily functions, including metabolism, immune response, and most especially, the body's response to stress.

Cortisol is basically the antithesis of what testosterone is. When in excess, Cortisol kills your positive hormones, causing long-term detriments to your body. To understand this, let's take a moment to look at how your body works.

Your body operates in a balance called homeostasis. Homeostasis is the body's process of maintaining internal stability, keeping factors like temperature, blood pressure, and pH within healthy ranges despite changes in the external environment.

We used the metaphor of a leaky ship to paint a picture of an unhealthy body. Similarly, a healthy body is like a perfectly ballasted ship, able to float above all the troubled waters of life. However, when you are dealing with a high-stress environment for extended periods of time, that's like sailing into a hurricane force gale again and again. It takes a toll on the ship!

Unfortunately, people often brush off the signs of stress, writing off the science with things like,

"Oh, I'm getting older,"

"Oh, this is just a part of life,"

"Oh, this is just how things are,"

It's not. I know this because I was there. I ignored the warning signs until I decided to make a change. Here's the thing, this is not just about police work. Sitting in front of a desk all day and typing on the computer can be a high stress environment. Any environment that always causes stress is detrimental to your hormone levels.

Military, first responders, caregivers, of course they will have a worsening hormone profile than a lot of other careers, but stress is still the primary killer in America. Stress is killing you. It's literally killing you, slowly, every day, like a death by a thousand papercuts.[17]

Just being in your home can do this.

One day, we had twin brothers come into the clinic — neither were military, police, or anything like that. They both worked normal jobs. They were genetically identical individuals but had *great variance in their hormone levels.* One was at much higher risk for illnesses than the other. What was going on?

Well, one of these brothers had three young children. There it is! That's stressful!

The sailing boat that was his body had three leaks in it, and he was starting to sink. Obviously, the kids themselves weren't the problem (no way!), but how he was dealing with the *stress* of those three kids (he was *not* dealing with it), was.

Your body has a natural ballast point. You can tell when you're in this homeostasis. The signals are: you're able to sleep, you're able to function sexually, you're able to feel that you're enjoying life.

When you're not, you're not.

However, not all stress is bad. In fact, small amounts of it are good for you. Brief, controlled stress strengthens both body and mind, a process known as *hormesis.* It's the same principle behind why grapes that endure a little hardship during the growing season produce the richest, most complex wines.

---

[17] Morgan, Charles A., Gary A. Hazlett, Gary L. Wang, and Gregory M. Southwick. 2000. "Stress-Induced Hormone Alterations in Special Operations Soldiers: The Impact of Stress on Hormonal Responses." *Psychoneuroendocrinology* 25 (5).

The antithesis of this is that running away from stress, pretending it isn't there, doesn't save you; it destroys you. Chronic stress has been linked to some of the biggest killers in America today. We're talking cardiovascular disease, diabetes, depression, immune dysfunction, even accelerated cognitive decline. You name it. If you let stress run wild, it eats away at your body from the inside out. Studies have shown that prolonged stress literally reshapes the brain and primes you for chronic disease.[18] That's the cost of not facing it head-on.

Hardship is resistance training, and the muscle it builds is your brain. Sound familiar? The same rule keeps appearing: **lean into the hurt to get to the healthy**. But how do we distinguish between the hurt of positive stress and the pain of constant stress?

BEYOND THE BADGE

I want to make this clear, if your career is military, police, etc., I am not telling you to leave your profession. However, I am telling you that you must understand the conse-quences of that profession. If you are in these fields, you need to do everything you can to optimize your *lifestyle* before your profession shortens your *lifespan*.

This starts by being informed. The good news is, there's hope. I'm going to take you step by step through the process of stress-healing using the hard knock lessons I went through: stress, breaking point, and taking action.

---

[18] McEwen, Bruce S. 1998. "Protective and Damaging Effects of Stress Mediators." *New England Journal of Medicine* 338 (3): 171–79.

STRESS SIGNALS

I was in my late 20s. I worked midnight shifts from 10:00 PM to 8:00 AM, Thursday night, Friday night, and Saturday night, and then a double shift on Sundays, working from 3:00 PM to sometimes as late as 2:00 AM.

The woman I was with at the time would wait up for me so that we could watch TV together. One night, she told me that I had spent the whole hour not watching the TV, but staring at the wall. I would have a blank stare on my face 'like I was looking into the void of outer space.'

I don't remember staring at the wall. What I do remember is what extreme stress feels like. Those were the signals my body was sending, and I ignored every one of them. Let me give you a lighter-hearted example.

I remember coming home late one night, and I ate an entire bucket of ice cream. Not the little baby bucket. I'm talking the big bucket. 3000 calories worth of ice cream! It was vanilla bean.

Hindsight is 20/20. What I didn't know at the time was that I was looking for some kind of comfort. I was trying to process a tremendous amount of stress and didn't know it. Many men and women that are in truly dangerous professions will run and hide from their own stress, under the false assumption that by doing so they are protecting themselves and their people. I never told my partner what I was going through. I thought that I was protecting her by doing so.

Look, we all need time to process what we go through, and sometimes we need to do that alone. I get that. For me, a vital outlet was the gym. With exercise, I was able to focus my negative energy into a positive outlet. Energy doesn't just dissipate or go away. Energy is used. It can be used for a negative action or a positive action.

So, you're either going to direct that negative energy into eating ice cream, ignoring your spouse, and being depressed, or you're going to divert it into, "Hey, I'm going to take this action, I'm going to build the best body that I can, and I'm going to do something healthy with the energy that I have."

THE NIGHT SHIFT SHOOTOUT

This really happened during one of my midnight shifts.

I'd moved from Cleveland PD to the Clearwater Police Department in Florida. It was very close to Christmas, and it was my last night in post-academy, so I had a field training officer with me. We got a call for a potentially disturbed male. Whatever, this happens a thousand times, nothing to write home about… Right?

We rolled up to this home that had a front patio breezeway. I told my training officer and two other cops, "Stay behind concealment. I'm going to run up, knock on the door, and come back out."

I run up, knock on the door, come back out, and start peeking around the corner of the breezeway. I see the bad guy. He's walking by, holding a long rifle with two pistols in his pocket, and a shotgun on his back.

I said to myself, "Well, that's interesting…"

He's hunting for us. I knew there was a young kid in the house, because he was the one that had called us. So, now we were in a very *stressful* situation. Soon, we have cops everywhere around this house. And we're searching for him as he's hunting for us.

I'm now on the corner of the house next door, and what I don't know is – he's walking between houses right towards me. I just started to lean my head past the corner when I heard a shot ring out. Then, two other officers immediately fired.

Suddenly, I was ripped back.

Someone had grabbed the handle on my bullet proof vest and pulled me away from the corner just as the shots rang out. I fell flat on my butt. I'm 240lbs of muscle, and I'm standing tactically, so how the hell did I fall on my butt?

The suspect was taken down, and later, during our after-action report (where we gather to give our statements), I'm asking, "Hey, who pulled me back?"

My buddies tell me, "What are you talking about? You fell on your butt!"

"No, I didn't. Somebody pulled me back — I was at the corner of the house completely *alone*."

Was it God or a guardian angel that saved me? I have no clue what it was, but I do know that I'm alive for a reason. This was not the first or the last time that I've felt God's presence on my shoulders during my life's most stressful moments.

Stress is a God-given tool for our bodies to overcome our greatest challenges. It's for the death-valleys of life, not our day to day. Knowing the difference may save your life.

SEE THE SIGNS. TAKE CONTROL.

What stress is for you will be particular to you. For me, I started noticing the signs of stress when I became depressed. I'm not a depressed person, but found myself gaining belly fat, feeling unmotivated, and with a lowered sex drive. I asked myself, "What the heck is going on? I'm healthy, I do all the exercise I can do…"

Were the tubs of ice cream not a great additive? Sure. But was that making me fat with the amount that I was working out? Nope. There was some other cause. What was my sex drive like? Almost nonexistent. Period. I was sluggish. I had constant brain fog. Something needed to change. This was not the life I wanted to live.

Because I'd taught myself so much about hormones already, I knew what the next best step to take was. I went to my healthcare clinic to get my testosterone levels checked. I was at 600 nd/L. From over 1,400 at my peak, I was now halfway to the bottom.

You know what my doctor said?

"Yeah, Tomo, you're fine."

"Fine? Doc, no I'm not! It's literally half of what I'm supposed to be!"

"Well, the chart says… blah blah blah…"

In all seriousness, I'm grateful for what my doctor said. It forced me to seek out alternative methods for my healthcare. I sought out a rejuvenation clinic that understood how to treat hormones properly.

I say this to all my patients: I was a patient first. I understand the failings of the healthcare system because the healthcare system *failed me*. The failure is this: They are not examining the root cause of our problems. If I would have just followed that doctor's cadence, told him I was depressed, got on weight loss pills and antidepressants, I would not be living the best life I am today.

SHORTCUTS CUT YOUR LIFE SHORT

Big medicine has brainwashed us into thinking that there's a pill for every ill. People don't think there's anything wrong with their stress or depression treatments because the medical system is not telling them anything's wrong.

Big Medicine is telling us, "Oh you have high cholesterol? Here's some statin for that!"

"Oh, this statin is now giving you high blood sugar? Keep taking your statin!"

"Oh, your statin is no longer working, and now you have type-II diabetes? Here's some metformin and insulin!"

We can see the consequences of this very clearly now. If your medications are only masking your issue, then your issue is still slowly killing you. Remember, stress kills you. It's a death by a thousand paper cuts, and stress pills are like little

Band-Aids. It might be *sopping* up the bleeding, but it's not *stopping* the bleeding.

I want to be clear for those that are feeling angry with me right now. Mental health medications have their place. I've mentioned that before. But think about this:

If you're on depression medication because you're at risk of suicide, and a side-effect of your medication is suicide, are you not ultimately treating your suicide with suicide?[19]

My advice is this: **Optimize your life before you cut your life short with a shortcut.**

No doctor wants you to be sick. But because they've been taught to only treat things with a pill for every ill, they're unintentionally exacerbating the illnesses they're trying to cure. Having depression, and I say this very carefully, is largely a misdiagnosis for *most* people. Treat your situation first by optimizing your lifestyle; if that doesn't fix it, then treat your hormones; if *that* doesn't fix it, then it's chemical or genetic issue, and that's where the industry has its place.

Honestly, it should be *criminal* to not make sure a patient has checked their major biomarkers before putting them on a medication whose symptom is suicide. It's malpractice. Basic science says that your body can't work properly without adequate hormone levels. So, why aren't mainstream medicine and psychotherapy — the medicine of the mind — checking hormone levels first?

---

[19] Reeves, R. R. "Antidepressant Induced Suicidality: An Update." *Psychiatry (Edgmont)* 7, no. 12 (2010): 42–46.

BRINGING IT ALL TOGETHER

Everybody's going to go through some sort of stress crisis in their life, probably much more than once. It doesn't matter if you're a cop, a soldier, or an insurance salesman. If you don't face up to your stressors, your stress will face you, and you'll lose, little by little. You're going to crash at some point too, based on age. Menopause and andropause are coming. Are you ready for it?

You can either have a negative cascading effect (stress compounding stress) or a positive cascading effect (optimization compounding optimization). The choice is yours to make. There are tools, methodologies, and ways of being and acting that ensure your body processes things correctly, so that you can go forward in the cycle of becoming well. When is the best time to start?

Yesterday.

I don't say this to scare you, but the cost of not optimizing your life is your life. Your health is your life. The opposite of that is death. Yes, the cliché is true: We are all, in fact, slowly dying. That's no reason for despair or inaction. How well you want to live the life you have is completely up to you. As for me, I believe that **optimizing our health is the most unselfish thing we can do as human beings.**

Why?

Because we don't live longer for ourselves. We live longer for those we love, for our family, for our community, our country, and our world. Just like within our very bodies, *we* are not just isolated atoms. We exist in a holistic continuity of life and lives. Living healthy makes all that lives around us healthier too.

If you're skeptical of that claim, listen to this. I've said this before, but I want to reiterate it here, because this point is very important:

I want to *run* with my kids and grandkids when I'm 67 years old. I have people that are my age, 40 years old, that are damn near crippled. They're overweight. They have no energy. Do you think that their lifestyle is a healthy life model for their children?

Absolutely not.

Do you think that modelling a healthy lifestyle will make our children into healthy, happy, and even wealthy individuals?

Absolutely. 100%. (Ronnie Coleman voice) Yea, buddy!

This system that I am guiding you through, *Operation Optimal*, works. I know it works because it worked for me. I have more energy now at 40 than I ever did at 30 or even 25 years old. And you don't have to be a bodybuilder like me to feel as good as I do!

I know *Operation Optimal* works because it's *working* for thousands of individuals that come through my clinic. The best part is, you don't have to come through my clinic to optimize your life. You just have to apply the daily principles and knowledge that this book guides you on.

If this sounds exciting to you, and I hope it does, you can download my free *Health Optimization Guide* at the QR code below. It condenses this entire book into a weekly, repeatable action plan. There are pages in there for you to journal, reflect, and even collaborate on your health journey with other like-minded individuals. There's also a printed guide I can ship directly to your door for just $10 total.

Your life is made up of many days. A healthy day becomes a healthy, wealthy, and happy life sooner than you think. Go to the QR code to start optimizing your life day-by-day today!

CHAPTER 5

Become your Body's Best Expert

Have you ever taken a test and the teacher lets you bring in a one-page cheat sheet?

That's what this chapter is about – except this time, the test is your physical health, the classroom is your doctor's office, and the cheat-sheet is a *challenge-sheet* that equips you with essential knowledge, empowers you to push back on your doctor's assumptions and biases (and maybe your own too), and teaches you how to be informed on that most important of all subjects, YOU!

What if you could walk into your yearly physical more informed about *you* than your doctor? This should be the norm, but it sounds like the exception. Your body is you. It's not a holy mystery for the high priests to reveal. It's your history, your numbers, your risk factors, and your questions.

Your goal should be to walk into the exam room with confidence, context, and the ability to challenge surface-level assumptions. Most people don't do this. They walk in blindly.

They accept whatever gets prescribed to them, and the cycle of *a pill for every ill* starts from there.

But when you understand the game, what's being tested, what isn't, and why, you stop being a passive patient and start being your own advocate. You become your body's best expert. This chapter is designed to help you become just that.

THE MINIMUMS OF STANDARD TESTING

Before we can talk about what doctors should be testing for, let's look at what they actually test for.

When you go in for your yearly checkup, most doctors order a few basic tests. Think of these like the "standard package" on a car, just the essentials, nothing fancy. Here's what that usually includes:

CBC (COMPLETE BLOOD COUNT)

This test looks at the main parts of your blood — red blood cells, white blood cells, and platelets. It's like taking inventory of your body's delivery trucks (red cells), security guards (white cells), and repair crew (platelets). It helps find issues like infections or anemia, but it only gives a surface-level view of your health.

CMP (COMPREHENSIVE METABOLIC PANEL)

This one checks about 14 different things in your blood, including liver and kidney function, blood sugar, and electrolytes. Picture it like running a systems check on your car's engine — it tells you if things are running too hot, too low, or out of balance. It's helpful, but still broad.

Depending on your age and sex, your doctor might add a few more:

TSH (THYROID STIMULATING HORMONE)

This test measures how well your thyroid, your body's "metabolism thermostat", is working. But here's the problem: most doctors stop there. TSH is only one gear in a much bigger machine. Without checking the rest of the thyroid hormones, they're guessing what's wrong based on one dial reading. We'll come back to this later.

CHOLESTEROL PANEL

This test measures fats in your blood, things like LDL (bad cholesterol), HDL (good cholesterol), and triglycerides. It helps predict heart health. But most doctors only look at your total cholesterol, which is like judging a football team by the final score without knowing who actually played well or who blew the game.

PSA (PROSTATE-SPECIFIC ANTIGEN)

This one's for men. It measures a protein from the prostate gland, and high levels can mean inflammation, enlargement, or possibly cancer. It's a great early warning sign. Unfortunately, some doctors still insist on following it up with that dreaded "finger test." If PSA gives you the information, why make it invasive?

And that's it. Most doctors stop there. That's not medicine. That's assembly-line diagnostics. It's what insurance allows and prefers because it's quick to read, cheap to run, and easy to prescribe from. A doctor will look at your results from these basic tests, see a red flag on the handout (it could be as simple as 201 on your cholesterol vs. 200), and have a prescription (statin) ready to go. So, the assembly line that is the yearly checkup goes something like this:

GENERIC TEST → RED FLAG → PRESCRIPTION → NEXT!

It happens quickly. Do you know how much time the average patient spends with their primary care provider? Just above twelve minutes.[20] Is that enough time for a truly whole-body analysis and discussion?

Hell no!

Patients *and doctors* agree with me on this. Doctors are not spending enough time with their patients. A recent study conducted by the University of Chicago, Johns Hopkins University, and Imperial College London, used a simulation to compute time per patient based on data from the National Health and Nutrition Examination Survey. They found that the average primary care provider would need **26.7 hours per day** to see their average number of patients *and provide them with the recommended care* following national guidelines.[21] There just isn't enough time in a day!

So, in summary, doctors are overworked, overprescribing, and undertesting – why is this the way that it is?

---

[20] Medscape. Medscape Physician Compensation Report 2017. New York: WebMD, 2017.

[21] University of Chicago Medical Center. "Primary Care Doctors Would Need More than 24 Hours per Day to Provide Recommended Care." *UChicago Medicine*, August 5, 2022.

Before we can answer that question, we need to do a quick biology lesson. Don't worry, I've kept this as simple as possible, giving you only what you need to know to become your body's best expert.

IT'S ALL ABOUT THE HORMONES

Your body runs on hormones, period. I don't care if you're a Fortune 500 CEO or living under a bridge, your entire system is dictated by hormones. If you're a man, you run mainly on testosterone. If you're a woman, you run mainly on estrogen and progesterone. Here's a summary of how your hormone system (called *the endocrine system*) works.

WHAT ARE HORMONES?

Hormones are your body's way of balance (homeostasis). They fine-tune the activity of your cells, speeding things up or slowing them down so your system stays in harmony. Think of it like the fuel in your car, but also the cruise control, making sure you're not red-lining or stalling out. Without hormones, there's no movement, no rhythm, no homeostasis, and without that balance, everything starts to break down.

HOW DO HORMONES WORK?

Your hormones are like messages your body sends to keep everything running smoothly, kind of like text messages between your brain and your organs.

It all starts in your brain, with two key players: the **hypothalamus** and the **pituitary gland**. The hypothalamus is the boss — it decides what messages need to go out. The pituitary is the messenger — it stores those hormones and sends them out when the hypothalamus gives the signal.

The crazy part? Your pituitary gland is no bigger than a pea, but it's one of the most powerful organs in your entire body. It's like the control tower at an airport, tiny, but in charge of directing traffic for everything else.

Your body makes more than fifty different hormones, but we're going to focus on just nine of the main ones. These include:

- **Four tropic hormones** that tell other glands what to do.

- **Three growth-related hormones** that act directly on specific organs.

- **Two hormones from the posterior lobe** that handle key body functions.

MEET YOUR HORMONES

Now that we know where hormones come from, let's talk about some of the main ones and what they actually *do*.

Think of each hormone like a worker with a specific job. Some manage stress, others control growth, and some even handle reproduction. Here's a quick rundown of your top nine:

TSH (THYROID-STIMULATING HORMONE)

This one's like your body's thermostat operator. It tells your thyroid to release hormones that control your metabolism and body temperature. In short, it helps keep your energy and development on track.

ACTH (ADRENOCORTICOTROPIC HORMONE)

This hormone knocks on the door of your adrenal glands — your built-in stress managers — and tells them to release steroids that help your body handle pressure and stay balanced. Think of it as the captain calling in reinforcements during tough times.

FSH (FOLLICLE-STIMULATING HORMONE)

This one teams up with LH to handle reproduction. For women, it helps eggs mature and prepares the body for ovulation. For men, it keeps sperm production steady. Basically, it's the fertility foreman.

LH (LUTEINIZING HORMONE)

LH works right beside FSH. In women, it triggers ovulation, the big event of the menstrual cycle. In men, it signals the testes to make testosterone. It's the hormone that makes sure the reproductive system stays on schedule.

GH (GROWTH HORMONE)

This is your body's builder. It helps your bones grow, your muscles strengthen, and your tissues repair. Think of GH as your body's construction crew, constantly rebuilding and upgrading your structure.

PROLACTIN

Prolactin is the milk-maker. It activates the mammary glands so mothers can breastfeed, one of the many ways the body knows exactly what to do when it's time to nurture new life.

MSH (MELANOCYTE-STIMULATING HORMONE)

This one talks directly to your skin cells, telling them to make melanin, the pigment that gives your skin its color. You can think of it as your body's natural sunshade manager.

OXYTOCIN

This is sometimes called the "bonding hormone." It causes muscles to contract — during labor, breastfeeding, and even moments of closeness or affection. It's what helps us connect physically and emotionally.

ADH (ANTIDIURETIC HORMONE)

This hormone manages your body's water balance. It tells your kidneys to hold onto water instead of sending it all out as urine. You can think of ADH as your body's hydration supervisor, making sure you don't run dry.

HOW DO HORMONAL GLANDS WORK?

Your hormones come from a network of glands spread throughout your body. Four of these glands are dedicated almost entirely to making hormones, while others pitch in to support the system. Let's break down the main players and what they do.

THYROID GLAND

Your thyroid sits at the base of your neck and looks a bit like a butterfly. Don't let its size fool you — it plays a massive role in how your body runs. It makes two main hormones, **T3** and **T4**, which influence everything from your energy levels to your heart rate. These hormones also help keep calcium in your bones, which is crucial for healthy growth in kids.

In short, your thyroid helps control:

- Your metabolism (how fast your body burns energy)

- Your body temperature

- How your body uses carbs and fats

- Reproductive health

- Heart function

You can think of the thyroid as your body's engine tuner — keeping everything humming at the right speed.

PARATHYROID GLANDS

Behind your thyroid are four tiny glands called the **parathyroids**. They control how much calcium stays in your blood. Calcium isn't just for bones — it's essential for your muscles to contract and for your nerves to fire properly. These little glands act like the thermostat for your body's calcium levels, constantly adjusting to keep the balance just right.

ADRENAL GLANDS

Your adrenal glands sit like little hats on top of your kidneys. They produce a mix of hormones that help you stay balanced and respond to stress.

- **Aldosterone** helps regulate salt, potassium, blood pressure, and blood volume — like the body's hydration and pressure control system.

- **Cortisol** is your main stress hormone. It manages how your body uses fat, protein, and carbs for fuel, and helps you stay calm and steady under pressure.

When your adrenals are working right, they're like a built-in survival kit — keeping you alert, balanced, and ready for whatever comes.

PINEAL GLAND

Deep in the center of your brain sits a tiny, pine-cone-shaped gland called the **pineal gland**. It produces **melatonin**, the hormone that helps you fall asleep and stay on a natural rhythm. Melatonin also supports body temperature, appetite, and even acts as an antioxidant, helping protect your cells from wear and tear.

You can think of the pineal gland as your internal nightlight. It tells your body when it's time to power down and rest.

Pancreas Your pancreas sits tucked between your stomach and your spine. It's part of both your digestive and hormonal systems, a two-in-one kind of organ. Its main job is to keep your blood sugar balanced by releasing two key hormones:

- **Insulin**, which lowers blood sugar after you eat.

- **Glucagon**, which raises blood sugar when it gets too low.

You can think of insulin and glucagon as teammates — one steps on the gas, the other hits the brakes — keeping your energy levels steady all day long.

OVARIES AND TESTES

These glands (you know where they are) make eggs in women and sperm in men. They also produce your main sex hormones — **estrogen** and **progesterone** for women, and **testosterone** for men.

These hormones don't just control reproduction. They affect things like your mood, energy, sex drive, muscle tone, and even how confident you feel. In short, they're a big part of what makes you *you*.

OTHER HORMONE PRODUCERS

Almost every organ in your body makes some kind of hormone — not just the glands we've talked about. Your **kidneys**, **heart**, **skin**, and **gut** all produce hormones that help them do their jobs. It's like each organ has its own mini lab, creating the chemical signals it needs to stay healthy and communicate with the rest of your body.

So, **in conclusion**, hormones are as complex as they are important. That was a lot of information to take in, and believe me, that was the absolute basics! Now, look at all that complexity and compare it to the basic, run-of-the-mill blood test you get from your primary care… See the problem?

Most physicians will run a **CBC** (Complete Blood Count), **CMP** (Comprehensive Metabolic Panel), lipid panel, and TSH (Thyroid-Stimulating Hormone Test), and maybe throw in estradiol if you press them. But that's barely scratching the surface.

It would be like your local mechanic glancing at the idiot light on your dashboard and making a repair based on that. That's it. No looking under the hood or chassis. No full-scale diagnostic. Just a blinky red light and, "Hey, you need a new transmission! That'll be five grand please!"

If that approach is not good enough for your *car*, why is it good enough for your actual body!?

In this next section, I'll tell you what a real, full-scale clinical testing should look like and why it matters.

WHAT DOCTORS SHOULD TEST FOR

In addition to the bare minimum, to really understand what's driving your symptoms, we need to run a deeper systems panel. At minimum, that includes these three key areas:

1. **The Major Hormones**

2. **Thyroid Function**

3. **The Inflammatory Markers**

1. **MAJOR HORMONES:**

- Testosterone or Estrogen & Progesterone

    - You'll want to measure your Total, Free, and Bio-available levels of these.

    - Optimal values for these will vary depending on the individual, time of the month, time of the day, etc.

- FSH (Follicle Stimulating Hormone)

- LH (Luteinizing Hormone)

- Pregnenolone

    - This is the master hormone; it works as a precursor to many others

- SHBG (Sex Hormone Binding Globulin)

    - This binds hormones and affects their availability

- Estradiol

    - Check for both men and women to measure estrogen and testosterone balance. These two hormones don't just operate in isolation' they work in a ratio that influences mood, energy, muscle development, fat distribution, and even long-term health markers. If one outweighs the other too much, you'll feel it in your performance and daily life. Balance is the key, because it keeps the entire system stable and functioning the way it's supposed to.

- Progesterone

  - This is especially important for women, and women are the only ones usually tested for it.

- PSA (Prostate-Specific Antigen)

  - This applies only to men. Get this checked before a finger goes up the bum.

These hormones are your day-to-day hormones, the ones that really affect what we call symptoms. And they're also rarely tested, even if you ask.

2. THYROID FUNCTION

Your thyroid doesn't work alone: it responds to orders from the pituitary gland. These labs help determine if your thyroid is actually doing its job, not just how much TSH is yelling at it.

Test for:

- TSH (Thyroid Stimulating Hormone)

- Free T3

- Free T4

- Reverse T3

- Thyroid Antibodies

  - This is especially critical for women with autoimmune tendencies

3. INFLAMMATORY MARKERS

These are your silent saboteurs. High inflammation doesn't always show up with pain, but it will show up later as heart disease, autoimmunity, or fatigue. Catch it early. All of these are upstream indicators of heart disease, autoimmune issues, and chronic fatigue.

- CRP (C-Reactive Protein)
  - Marker of systemic inflammation; elevated in chronic disease and infection.

- Homocysteine
  - Amino acid linked to heart disease and stroke risk when elevated.

- Ferritin
  - Protein that stores iron; high or low levels indicate inflammation and/or deficiency.

4. ADDITIONAL MARKERS

These labs give you further insight into metabolic function, insulin sensitivity, and long-term aging risk. In a real optimized health panel, they should be non-negotiable.

- Insulin
  - Hormone that regulates blood sugar; elevated levels signal insulin resistance and metabolic dysfunction.

- IGF-1 (Insulin-like Growth Factor)
  - Growth hormone marker tied to aging, recovery, and longevity.

- LDL Particle Size

  - This refers to the diameter of low-density lipoprotein particles, which are a type of cholesterol carrier in the blood.

  - Breaks down LDL into large (safer) or small (more harmful) particles; better predictor of heart risk than total LDL.

If you're not testing these, you're not looking for the cause, you're just reacting to the symptoms. This isn't luxury lab work. It's foundational health intelligence. It's what the *bare minimum* should be.

THE REAL REASON THIS IS MISSED

Here's the sad truth: Most general practitioners don't even know how to interpret this kind of data. They're not trained in it. They might push you to a specialist. They might say, "You don't need it."

They might flat-out refuse.

Why? Because their job isn't to optimize your health. It's to keep you within the "normal" range. But what is normal? "Normal" on a lab chart means "average." And the average man today is overweight, stressed, and hormonally depleted.

So, what happens when your testosterone is 450? Your doctor shrugs. "That's within range."

But guess what? Your grandfather's average was 900! You feel like crap. But it's "normal." So, no help. Or, let's get you on the *pill for every ill* cycle, and you have the negative cascading effect, and so on.

This problem is why the *Tomo Challenge Sheet* exists – to help you push back! Think of it as your personal health dossier. When you go into the doctor's office, all you need to do is **ask three simple questions**.

THE TOMO CHALLENGE SHEET

1. WHAT ARE YOU TESTING AND WHY?

Ask: "Hey Doc, what are you testing me for today?"

Follow-up: "And why are you testing those things?"

Challenge: "Hey Doc, are there any other markers we should look at to get a clearer picture?"

2. WHAT ARE YOU *NOT* TESTING AND WHY NOT?

Ask: "Are you checking *all* my hormone levels?"

Follow-up: "Hey Doc, are we testing thyroid function beyond just TSH?"

Challenge: "Can we include inflammatory markers?"

3. WHAT'RE MY OPTIONS *BEFORE* MEDICATION?

Ask: "If my numbers are off, what are the root causes?"

Follow-up: "Are there lifestyle changes that would fix this instead of medication?"

Challenge: "Doc, what are the symptoms that go along with the pill you're prescribing?"

The point of the challenge sheet is to reframe the doctor-patient relationship. You're not there to be managed. You're there to be informed. Remember, your doctor is there to serve you.

WHEN THE DOCTOR PUSHES BACK

When you ask these questions, most doctors will say:

"You don't need that."

"Your levels are fine."

"That's not how we do it."

"Your insurance doesn't cover that."

Your reply should be something like:

"Doc, how do you know I don't need it if you haven't tested me for it? If this is about insurance coverage, I'll pay out of pocket. I want answers."

And if they still won't budge?

Fire them. I'm serious! Find a better doctor!

A good doctor is your partner in health, not your warden. If they're not on board with understanding the full picture, they're not the right doctor for you.

HOW TO THINK CRITICALLY WITHOUT OVERTHINKING

We've covered a lot of ground in this chapter, and it's long for a reason: This is the marrow of the book. But I wouldn't be doing my job if I gave you all this info about your body without telling you how to think about yourself *for yourself.*

There's a right way and a wrong way to do research. **And most people are doing it wrong.**

THE WRONG WAY

Google a symptom. Fall into a subreddit. End up buying snake oil from some guy who read a headline once and now thinks he's a health guru. That's not research. That's how people get stuck in loops of confusion, fear, and misinformation.

The other extreme is just as bad. Take a flu shot every year. Jab in every vaccine under the sun. Get on as many antidepressants as you can carry. That's not *trusting the science*. That's how people become sheep and end up compromising on their long-term health and wellness for nothing.

Both of these extremes are dysfunctional.

Most people research from a biased perspective based on what they were told their entire life in science class or from TV commercials. That's not research. That's programming.

This is why men end up blocking their DHT just to keep their hairline intact and then wonder why they feel like sh#t!

Blocking DHT to stop hair loss is nuts. That's the hormone that makes you a man. You want to look healthy and bald or unhealthy and hairy? Pick one!

THE RIGHT WAY

Learn how the body works when it's perfect. Remember, your body is a perfectly running machine. That's the idea that you build from. Learn what your body does when it's healthy, when it's operating exactly how it's supposed to. That's the baseline. You don't start with what's broken. You start with how it was designed to function.

You can use Google if you want. You can use ChatGPT. You can use whatever. But those aren't sources. Those are search tools. Know how your tool works before you use it. Each one has its own bias and agenda. Mainstream medicine is a symptom-treatment enterprise. It's there for money. Big Pharma wants to sell you a pill. Conspiracy influencers want to sell you distrust. Both sides have motives.

So don't just take a headline and run with it. Don't just take what I say and run with it. Ask real questions. Interrogate the data. Look for the mechanism behind the claim. Does it follow logic? Is it consistent with what a healthy body should be doing?

You've got to ask: How does the human body work? What is the perfect version of this perfect machine? What should this system be doing when it's not messed up by years of stress, bad food, and bad information?

Here's what I recommend.

1. Go get an anatomy book. Look up what hormones do. Find out what signals what. Your body is all interconnected to itself.

2. Ask questions. What do peptides do? What causes a cascade? What is a cascade? What turns this or that on and off. Don't just look for solutions to your symptoms. Look for the source of the problem.

Once you've got a handle on what the body is supposed to do, you can start tracking what's not happening, and do it logically.

For example, the hypothalamus talks to the pituitary. The pituitary signals your testes (or ovaries) to produce testosterone (or estrogen/progesterone). Those are sex hormones that affect your energy, mood, sleep, and metabolism. So if you're falling off somewhere downstream, let's say your sex drive is low or you're depressed, go upstream. Okay, I found out my testosterone is low. Now let's go further upstream and find out why pituitary is not signaling properly, and so on.

You fix the system by understanding the system. Good research isn't just about facts. It's about questions. It's about knowing what to ask and where to look for the answer.

This is how you stop reacting to symptoms and start hunting down root causes. You're not looking for a pill. You're looking for the breakdown in the chain. That's why *Operation Optimal* exists. Not to scare you. Not to sell you. To inform you and help you take back control over what matters most.

ACTION STEPS

1. BRING THE TOMO CHALLENGE SHEET TO YOUR NEXT PHYSICAL

Don't walk into your doctor's office unarmed. Print the challenge sheet and keep it in your medical folder. Ask what they're testing, what they're not testing, and why. If your doctor gives you pushback, don't fold, push back. If they get mad at you, tell them to get mad at me instead! I can take the heat!

2. BUILD YOUR BASELINE KNOWLEDGE WITH REAL LEARNING

Before you Google a symptom, study how your body works when it's not broken. Go to the library or order a real physiology or endocrinology test. Highlight how the hormone cascade functions, how signaling works, and how upstream problems lead to downstream symptoms. Use this as your foundation.

3. REVERSE-ENGINEER ONE SYMPTOM YOU'VE BEEN IGNORING

Pick one thing you've been dealing with: fatigue, low sex drive, stubborn weight, poor sleep, and trace it upstream. What hormone systems affect it? What markers should be tested? Which lab numbers relate to it? Write out your hypothesis, then schedule bloodwork (with a willing provider or third-party lab) to confirm or challenge your theory. Treat it like a real investigation because your body deserves real answers.

CHAPTER 6

Knowing Your Optimal & How to Get There

OPTIMAL SHOULD BE NORMAL

One of my goals with this book is to help you get to your ideal state of body, mind, and spirit. So, now that we've learned about hormones in general, what is the optimal hormone level for you?

Nobody knows!
That's **the problem** we're facing.

Why does nobody know? Because nobody was testing their hormone levels at a young age, when you're at the most optimal level. Your optimal level of health is you at the peak of your health, usually around the age of 25.

Unless your hormones were tested at that age, there's no way for you to know what your optimal levels are right away. For example, when I was 19 years old, my testosterone levels were 1470 ng/dcl. That was my optimal. It is still my optimal. 1470 is the level I should be at today at 40 years old. That level is *off the charts* for most doctors, and most doctors will be concerned by that because it's not *normal*. They're wrong because normal is determined by the average. If we are in the midst of a declining hormone crisis, and we are, then *normal* is a race to the bottom.[22]

That's why this chapter is going to teach you how to determine and maintain the hormone profile that's optimal for you. Your normal should be your ideal.

OPTIMAL IS INDIVIDUAL

Everybody's body **is different.**

Your optimal hormone level will be unique to you. A testosterone level of 1470 nanograms per deciliter, or an estradiol level above about 400 pg/mL per milliliter, is far too much for most people. It would throw your body out of the delicate balance of homeostasis. So, what's the right amount for you?

A good hormone therapy clinic or clinician will find that answer carefully, methodically, and safely. At Aspire Rejuvenation, we start low and go slow. We titrate to the effect. We know someone has low testosterone or estrogen based on their symptoms. We up their hormone levels steadily until the symptoms disappear and they start feeling again how

---

22 Pataky, Miklós W., et al. "Hormonal and Metabolic Changes of Aging and the Acute to Chronic Adaptation." *Frontiers in Endocrinology* 12 (2021).

they were at their ideal age. 700 ng/dLel could be the point at which symptoms vanish and optimization begins. For others, like me, 700 ng/dLel would crash me out and give me every negative symptom out there.

My optimal is different than yours. Yours is different than mine. One is not *better* than the other. It's about what's *best* for you.

Your genetics play a part in this, along with the size of your body, the amount of fat and muscle mass you have, how your lifestyle is, how much sleep you get; all are factors that a good clinic and clinician will use to determine your optimal level. Later in this chapter, we'll discuss how to find a clinic or clinician if hormone optimization is right for you. First, I'd like to go into further detail about a particular type of hormones, the ones that're most relevant to your day-to-day.

SEX HORMONES ARE YOUR LIFE

In the last chapter, we did a general overview of all the hormones in your body, what they do, why they're there, and why they matter. All of your hormones are important, but it is your sex hormones that deeply affect your libido, your mentality, and your daily life. Optimizing your sex hormone levels is also optimizing your life. Let's break that down point by point in more detail, focusing on the effect of our sex hormones on our mentality.

YOUR SEX HORMONES DETERMINE YOUR GENDER

Unfortunately, this is a controversial thing to say nowadays! The fact is, if you have more testosterone, you are more masculine, both physically and mentally. If you have more estrogen, you are more feminine, physically and mentally.

Puberty makes this clear and obvious. During puberty, a boy turns into a man. What's one of the first things we notice when this happens? He starts having manly behaviors! Usually, these manly behaviors are not controlled well because they're occurring for the first time. We see things like uncontrolled aggressiveness, dominance, and wild libido.

For women, puberty shows up not only in female sex characteristics but also in feminine attitudes like emotional influx, heightened sensitivity to relationships, and stronger mood swings tied to hormonal shifts.

Sex hormones determine your sex. Your sex shapes your mentality.

SEX HORMONES SHAPE YOUR MENTALITY

Your mentality is *how you think*. We used puberty to show how an influx of hormones changes you. Now, we'll demonstrate how an *ebbing* of hormones affects you. With both of these examples, we can start to paint a picture of how your sex hormones affects your mental life.

When andropause and menopause occur, your hormones drop to very low levels. What happens to you mentally? You start to misunderstand how you're feeling and how you're thinking. The way that your brain works changes. You start to become depressed because *your brain runs on sex hormones.* You can even start to exhibit symptoms similar to psychosis, clinical depression, and even identity crisis. You may even start to question your ideas, morals, principles, and even your religious convictions! [23]

All of this shows that hormones don't just run your body; they shape the very lens through which you see yourself and the world.

THE PSYCHOLOGY AND CULTURE OF HORMONES

I'm excited to share this topic with you because this also serves as a preview for another book I will publish in the future!

We all know that there's a cultural element to masculine vs. feminine. From the war of the sexes, to that old *Gillette* controversy, to Sydney Sweeney in tight Levis, we are all aware of what the "Culture War" is. What if this culture war, and its congruent political divide, derives in some way from how our hormones have changed?

Our hormones are, after all, in crisis. We are plum-meting to the bottom, while our physical and mental health symptoms are rising like a flood. As our hormone levels have changed, so too has our culture.

This is not just correlation.

Books like *EstroGeneration* by Dr. Anthony G. Jay have linked our collective crisis of weight-gain, depression, infertili-ty, and other problems to the continuous exposure of our bod-ies to a class of chemicals called *estrogenics*, affecting both

---

[23] Gordon, Jessica L., and Hadine Joffe. "Depression, Menopause, and the Role of Hormone Therapy." *Medical Clinics of North America* 107, no. 1 (January 2023): 107–124.

men and women to cause earlier and earlier puberty rates and increasing feminization across the spectrum.

Let me say this before you attack me, **femininity is valuable** and essential to us as human beings, both culturally and biologically. However, femininity without a corresponding balance of *masculinity* is just as harmful to us as too much masculinity without a balance in femininity. **Our culture, just like our bodies, exists in homeostasis**. Disrupt the balance, and the culture sickens and dies.

Why are men not men anymore? There are men out there who's DHT levels are so low, they can't grow facial hair. Not even one follicle! Similarly, there are more and more men who are coming out as bisexual, homosexual, and transgender. While these are natural (albeit rare and fringe) lifestyles, we're seeing an unnatural increase in the frequency with which these things are occurring, and they're beginning at a younger and younger age. I'll leave some of my thoughts on this, particularly regarding hormone therapy for underage 'transgender' children for the next chapter. My point here is that **there is a demonstrable and causal trend between hormone decline, cultural change, and sexual expression**.[24]

If a boy is growing up with more feminine inundation hormones, and he's seeing more feminine dominance in his culture, of course he will have a tendency to grow up more

---

[24] Travison, Thomas G., Andre B. Araujo, Amy B. O'Donnell, Varant Kupelian, and John B. McKinlay. "A Population-Level Decline in Serum Testosterone Levels in American Men." *The Journal of Clinical Endocrinology & Metabolism* 92, no. 1 (January 2007): 196–202.

feminine. What's not obvious is how that's changing his brain chemistry, brain development, and his sexual orientation.

Is that boy ever really hitting the peak of his puberty? Is he reaching an optimal level of testosterone as determined by his genetics? Probably not.

Therefore, the level of our optimal hormones is also declining. We are losing our sense of what's normal and what's optimal for our young men, both physically and culturally. There's a price we're paying for that.

Suicide rates among young men are very alarming. In 2022, the suicide rate for males aged 15–24 was approximately 21.1 per 100,000, compared with only 5.8 per 100,000 for females in the same age group. Overall, males in 2023 accounted for nearly **80% of all suicides** despite comprising about half the population, with a male suicide rate around four times higher than that of females[25].

What effect does our culture have on these suicide rates? What effect do our hormones have on the hyper-feminization of our culture? The data on this is difficult to acquire, scandalizing to share, but pioneering to explore. It's both a tremendous problem for our children, and a tremendous opportunity for positive change.

If you're interested in these and other topics, I publish a weekly blog which you can subscribe to for free at:

tomomarjanovic.substack.com

---

[25] Centers for Disease Control and Prevention, Suicide and Self-Harm Injury: Data Brief No. 471, March 2024 (National Center for Health Statistics, 2024),

I hope to see you there and that you'll participate in the discussion, particularly if you disagree with me!

WHEN CONSIDERING HORMONE OPTIMIZATION

If you want to explore hormonal testing and optimization, but you feel overwhelmed or skeptical of the process and don't know where to start, here's my advice to you:

Start by getting the data.

Chapter 5 details what you should test for and what it means. If you can't get this information from your doctor, you can acquire it from a reputable hormone clinic. You don't have to come to Aspire Rejuvenation to do this. In fact, this book isn't an ad for me, so I'll say: *do not come into my clinic!*

I will however plug Summit Rejuvenation Center in St. Louis, MO. Their owner, Scott Otey, is both a great friend of mine and a great option for you if you live in the area.

Wherever you go, use the information I gave you in Chapter 5 to determine your hormone profile [go to pg. 75 for cheat sheet]

Once you have that data, you then need to decide what normal is and what your optimal should be. Do you feel normal? If you're tired all the time, depressed, and have low libido, that's not an acceptable definition of normal. Ask yourself these questions:

- How's my energy level?
- How do I sleep?

- What is my sex drive like?

- How's my mentality?

- What are my aches and pains like?

Don't accept negative answers to these questions as *normal* or as *just a part of the aging process*.

The average patient at our clinic is between 39 and 44 years old. That's when people start to have hormonal decline leading to detrimental symptoms. I've also seen patients with these problems as early as 35 to 25 years old. That's not *normal*. I encourage them to change their environment first and then, if that doesn't work, to change their hormones.

I offer that same advice to you:

If you are considering hormone therapy, **don't come to my clinic**.

Rather, **optimize your environment and lifestyle first**. You can utilize Chapter 3 of this book, my companion workbook, and the (coming soon) *Operation Optimal Rejuvenation Program* to get you in good health, wealth, and happiness the right way first. Fortunately, this book is the best possible introduction to all of these things!

If these actions do not work, or your life is already optimized in this way, and you are still suffering symptoms, then it's the right time for you to explore hormone therapy. I truly believe that everyone will need hormone optimization at some point in their lives, no matter how healthy you are, because aging and hormone decline is inevitable.

When that happens, here is how you can find a reputable clinic, know what to expect, and how to make it affordable and cost-effective.

HOW TO FIND HORMONE OPTIMIZATION: CLINICS & CLINICIANS

The most common response I hear from first-time patients after they undergo hormone optimization is something like this:

"Holy sh#t! I've never felt this good before! I've been missing this my entire life!"

If hormone therapy is right for you, and you want to feel this way, there are a few simple steps that you can take and pitfalls to look out for:

First, be wary of scams! There are a lot of money-grab clinics out there. They're male-focused, cookie cutter testosterone dispensaries. They're just as bad as the big-pharma medical establishment. Instead of a pill for every ill, it's testosterone with every meal. Everybody gets a peptide too! And then it's upsells, upsells, upsells. You're a dollar sign to them, not a person.

The way to avoid these scams is to **look for the clinic or clinician who treats you like an individual and tailors your treatment to you**. They will walk you through the process gradually and advise treatments based on your symptoms, not dollar signs. They will use the *minimal amount of intervention* to fix the problems that you have.

There are other telltale signs that you can use to distinguish a legitimate operation from a scam.

If you aren't talking to a doctor or a medical provider at some point during your consultation, such as only through a website, it's probably a scam. Rather, you should be face-to-face with an actual medical provider that is:

- Assessing you

- Looking through your medical chart

- Asking you *a lot of* questions

- Going through your blood work with you line by line

- Confirming what you're feeling

- Listening to your perspective

- Confirming what you're *not* feeling

- Discovering the things you didn't even realize were a problem

If these things are not happening in your experience with the clinic, get the f#ck away from that clinic!

Your body is a very delicate thing. Being prescribed too much testosterone, estrogen, or thyroid medication can cause serious problems like blood clots, liver damage, heart arrhythmia, mood disturbances, and increased risk of stroke.[26] Over-

---

[26] Mayo Clinic, "Hormone Therapy: Is It Right for You?" Mayo Clinic, last updated March 30, 2022

prescription of hormones is just as dangerous as with other medications. Would you trust just anyone to give you heart medication?

Hell no!

Bring that same mindset to bear as you seek out your hormone rejuvenation provider. Trust but verify.

Think about it like this. If you owned a Lamborghini (and I do recommend owning one at some point in your life!), would you take that Lamborghini into a Jiffy Lube for its maintenance? Probably not, and that's not a knock on Jiffy Lube! No, you'd take your Lamborghini to the people that made it, Lamborghini, to get it serviced. You take what's most precious to the experts to fix it.

Your body is more precious to you than any possession you could possibly own. Why don't we treat our bodies as the luxurious, invaluable, and most precious items that they are? Take your Lamborghini, your body, only to the experts.

HOW TO BUDGET FOR HORMONE OPTIMIZATION

Hormone optimization is not typically covered by most insurance plans. That's fine. Most insurance is a scam, along with the entire revolving door that is our healthcare industry (at least as it is in the US). I have no problem standing on the mountain top and screaming that.

Health insurance **is a scam!**

It was developed by Big Pharma to feed Big Pharma and Big Medicine. The same people that are a part of the FDA, who approve what drugs drug companies can use, are also executives in those some drug companies. Health insurance executives are also closely tied to these parties. It's all one big club, and you and I are not members! [27]

Without getting lost on a tangent, I would recommend *not even trying* to go through your insurance for your hormone optimization. Insurance will bill *just the lab* work at $2,000 to $3,000 dollars. I've seen wild numbers. They are not interested in helping you; they are interested in billing you.

Do you know how much a lab panel costs most patients when they go out of pocket at my clinic?

Less than $200.

That's right, an average hormone optimization screening should cost you only $200. Payment plans for that amount are also usually available. That is not a large sum when it comes to starting your health optimization journey with hormone therapy.

After your initial screening, your optimization program will typically cost **less than $100 a month**, beginning on a very low dosage with only one hormone infused, usually testosterone, estrogen, or progesterone. Extra infusions, like thyroid medication, will usually cost an extra **$100 dollars** a month per.

So, you should **budget for around $300-500 up front, and $100-$200 per month**. If you feel that amount is unaf-

[27] Kanter, Gabrielle P. "The Revolving Door in Health Care Regulation." *Health Affairs* 42, no. 3 (2023).

fordable, simply change your lifestyle to make it affordable. Cut the out-to-eat once a week, cut back on extraneous expenses, and explore payment plan options. Make it work. Your life, at least your *optimal* life, is what's at stake.

Health and wellness is not cheap, but it's more expensive to be sick. It's actually *too expensive* to be sick. Most hormone protocols begin to show tangible results in just 2-3 months. Once you are optimized, you can start living your best life on a trajectory towards wealth and lasting happiness. I've saved my advice for that trajectory for part three of this book!

Start optimizing your life *today* before it's too late *tomorrow*.

FAQS

---

1. **WHAT DOES "OPTIMAL" REALLY MEAN WHEN IT COMES TO HORMONES?**

   Optimal isn't the same as normal. Normal is based on the declining average in the population. Optimal means the unique levels at which *you* function best – your peak balance of health, energy, and mindset.

2. **HOW DO I KNOW WHAT MY OPTIMAL HORMONE LEVELS ARE?**

   Unless your hormone levels were measured when you were around 25 (your natural peak), you won't know your exact optimal right away. That's why a good clinician starts low, goes slow, and titrates until symptoms resolve.

3. **WHY ISN'T "NORMAL" A GOOD STANDARD TO GO BY?**

   Because normal is based on averages — and if the averages are dropping each generation, then "normal" is a race to the bottom. Optimal should be your true target, not normal.

4. **CAN MY OPTIMAL BE DIFFERENT THAN SOMEONE ELSE'S?**

   Absolutely. One person may thrive at 700 ng/dLel testosterone, while that level would wreck another. Genetics, body composition, lifestyle, and sleep all play a role in your unique optimal.

5. WHY ARE SEX HORMONES SO IMPORTANT?

Sex hormones like testosterone and estrogen are central to libido, mood, energy, mental clarity, and even identity. They don't just run your body; they shape the way you think and experience the world.

6. WHAT HAPPENS WHEN SEX HORMONES DECLINE DURING ANDROPAUSE OR MENOPAUSE?

As hormone levels drop, many people experience depression, confusion, mood swings, and even symptoms resembling psychosis or identity crisis. Hormones affect your brain chemistry as much as your body.

7. HOW DOES CULTURE TIE INTO HORMONES?

Hormones don't just shape individuals, they influence culture. Widespread hormonal decline has been linked to rising feminization, shifts in sexual expression, earlier puberty rates, and cultural polarization.

8. HOW DO I AVOID SCAM CLINICS?

Beware of cookie-cutter "testosterone mills" or online providers who never connect you with a real doctor. A legitimate clinic will review your blood work line by line, confirm your symptoms, and tailor a plan to you.

9. HOW MUCH SHOULD HORMONE OPTIMIZATION COST?

A lab panel should cost around $200 out of pocket, not thousands through insurance. Ongoing treatment typically runs $100–$200 per month. Budget intelligently, cut unnecessary expenses, and invest in your health.

10. SHOULD I TRY LIFESTYLE CHANGES BEFORE HORMONE THERAPY?

Yes. Always optimize your environment, diet, exercise, and sleep first. If symptoms persist despite these changes, that's when hormone therapy becomes the right step.

PART II

CHAPTER 7

Longevity &
The Next Generation

BLUE ZONES & ENVIRONMENTAL FACTORS

How long do you think you will live?

Let me rephrase the question, how long do you think you *could* live if you lived an optimal life, all your life?

To answer this question, let's take a look at Blue Zones. These are specific regions of the planet where populations experience exceptional longevity and vitality, living healthier lives with lower rates of chronic disease. Learning about these areas, what environmental factors are at play there, can give us an idea of how we should be living our lives, and how our longevity can be enhanced.

I like to call Blue Zones, *anti-aging zones*. These are zones where people are not aging like the rest of us are. For example, 80 years old is very old in the United States. Yet people in Japan are often 100 years old plus and still walking around briskly to buy fruit from the market. And who is the longest living demographic in the world? Japanese women![28]

The wildest thing about these anti-aging zones is that they all have wildly different diets and lifestyles. In other words, there's no one diet or way of living that makes you live longer. So, what's the common factor here? The common factor is that there is **a lack of toxins in their environments**, including certain electronics. There are things in our environ-ments in modern societies that are actively killing us!

Things like pollution, toxins in our water, GMOs, and processed foods. And the research is clear; these things are tied to higher rates of disease and shorter life expectancy.[29]

Can you minimize your exposure to these things if you're living in the modern world? Not completely.

So, what is our solution?

Looking again at these anti-aging zones, while they are all on different diets, the commonality to all these diets is **non-processed food**. We need real food. We need clean water. We also need less stress.

People that live in anti-aging zones are also very active. They move! They walk around and swim. Well, there's a reason for that: They have to fish; they have to hunt. They're not sedentary. None of these people are fat. Obesity is a luxury they simply can't afford.

---

[28] Eileen M. Crimmins, "Lifespan and Healthspan: Past, Present, and Promise," *The Gerontologist* 60, no. 6 (September 2020): 989–1001

[29] Leonardo Trasande, *Sicker, Fatter, Poorer: The Urgent Threat of Hormone-Disrupting Chemicals to Our Health and Future… and What We Can Do About It* (New York: Houghton Mifflin Harcourt, 2019)

In contrast, every problem that we have in our society today is based off of convenience:

- Fast food

- Drive-thrus

- Delivery apps

- Elevators and escalators instead of stairs

- Streaming and endless screen time instead of walking or playing outside.

These shortcuts are cutting our life short. The future of medicine is in prevention first. So, prevent things from happening by making sure that you're living a proper lifestyle. Learn from the long living!

It is a fact though that, however healthy we live, our modern environment is toxic. We can't ultimately escape that. This is where things like stem cells, exosomes, peptides, and a proper hormone profile come in. These are longevity-based treatments. They get you to the baseline of what we should be calling *normal*, the plateau where many people living in anti-aging zones already are.

I truly believe that, if we optimize properly, our ideal lifespan will be 120+ years old. Many of us will not face the dangers that our ancestors faced: war, famine, diseases. While this is still a reality of many people's lives (and that's a tragedy that should not happen in this modern world), if you're reading this book, these things will likely not affect you. More than likely, you have food in your pantry right now. What that means is that **you have the potential to live a longer, happier, and more fulfilled life.**

Imagine that living to 100 years old is just within your reach. Why not reach out and take it?

Not one of us can *know* when we will die. However, we can strive to live and love to the fullest. Personally, I've almost died several times already during my police career. It doesn't phase me anymore. Whenever I go, I go. In the meantime, I'll be doing everything I can to reach 120 years old, still feeling healthy and happy. I'll be seeing my great grandchildren running on the beach, and I hope to join in with them!

Call me optimistic or just call me optimal.

THE HORMONE CRISIS IN YOUTH

Let's move now to probably the most important topic of this chapter: our children. Our kids are simply not reaching their optimal hormone levels during puberty anymore.[30] What scientific innovations could reverse this generational decline, and should they be used preventively in younger populations?

A parent's responsibility is to take charge over their children's health. If children's health is in decline generationally, the solution to that problem is **not hormone therapy**. Unless there is a severe genetic or pituitary issue, children should nev-

---

[30] A. Abacı and Ö. Besci, "A Current Perspective on Delayed Puberty and Its Management," *Journal of Clinical Research in Pediatric Endocrinology* 16, no. 4 (2024): 379–400

er have to take hormone therapies for their wellness. These modalities are for an aging population to reach youthful optimization.

What is the solution then for this crisis?

It comes down to what parents are feeding their children's body, soul, and mind. So, what are parents in general feeding their children?

Toxicity.

Did you know that one in three children in America today will get Type II Diabetes?[31] It's appalling to me when I see a child who is obese or overweight. While many of our establishments and industries that provide food are partly to blame for this, there's no one *ultimately* to blame but the parents.

It's the parents' fault.

They give excuses like, "Oh, my kids won't eat anything but chicken nuggets."

Really? Your kid wants nothing but McNuggets? Okay, put real food in front of them. Put an actual grass-fed steak on their plate. Watch what happens.

My daughter, who's almost two years old at the time of this writing, will eat a steak right off the bone, using just her hands, and she's got the best jaw structure because of it. Her teeth are strong. She's very healthy.

If you're putting a steak, fresh vegetables, and healthy rice in front of your children and they still won't eat it, then send

---

[31] Urrutia-Rojas, Ximena, et al. "Prevalence of risk for type 2 diabetes in school children." *Journal of School Health* 76, no. 5 (May 2006): 189-194.

them to bed hungry. I'm serious! It's not abuse because guess what, the next morning, when they are hungry, they'll be begging you for that steak, whole eggs, and healthy foods.

The problem is that parents are giving children options. It is your responsibility as a parent to make sure your child understands how to be healthy. It is your responsibility to choose properly on behalf of your children.

Wouldn't children eat candy and doughnuts all day every day if they could? Is that the right choice for them?

The hormone crisis in our children is the result of the shortcuts we've made on diet, exercise, and even screen time. **Parents are lazy**. If you're a parent and that triggered you and you want to put this book down or throw it out the window — good!

I hope it gets you riled up because it might also motivate you to fix the problem. The best part is that you can fix it easily, your kids will thank you for it, and your family will be happier.

Here's the fix: **Set the right example for your kids.**

If parents live a ship-shape lifestyle, avoiding toxins, seed oils, inflammatory foods and other garbage, then their children will live like that too.

THIS APPLIES TO MENTAL DIET TOO

This same principle applies to our mental diet as well.

My daughter does not watch TV. My daughter does not have access to a phone. In fact, her mother and I will not even use our phone in front of our daughter. We don't want her to see us giving more attention to a screen than to her.

Using devices in front of our children tells them that the screen is more important than they are. That, in turn, will encourage them to believe that screens are more important than people. The iPad is today's babysitter. The iPad is today's, "Go play outside!"

This is very bad for children, and we won't know the full consequences of this until it's too late. Children are simply not ready for screens. It's causing actual brain damage to them because:

- They're being exposed to over-stimulation, a vibrancy of colors, sounds and interactivity

    - This causes a shortened attention span, hyperactivity, and poor emotional regulation

- They're being inundated with unregulated dopamine

    - This causes addictive behavior patterns, loss of interest in real-life play, early signs of anxiety and depression, and spoils their dopaminergic baseline

Now, because they've gotten so used to a screen with glowing lights and colors and sounds, they're not getting dopamine from simply being alive, looking at the leaves, or being in the sunshine. This is making our children unable to cope with or even appreciate reality.

This reconditioning carries over into adolescence. Why are teenagers, both boys and girls, but particularly young men, consuming pornography and being exposed and addicted to pornography at younger and younger ages?

Porn is the lazy and *convenient* alternative to socializing, wooing, and building a real relationship with a real person. The consequences of this shortcut is desocialization, desensitization, and a legion of mental health issues.[32] Convenience is the killer of society. Convenience is the killer of health. Convenience is the killer of wellness. It'll kill you. If you're taking shortcuts, it's actually killing you right now.

DOPAMINERGIC URGES

Dopamine is a chemical messenger in your brain that helps regulate mood, motivation, focus, and the feeling of reward. What drives you to take action and feel satisfaction when you achieve something, derives from dopaminergic urges and expression. We all, as pleasure-seeking beings, pursue dopaminergic release. In other words, we all want to feel good.

What we choose to feel good *from* is what separates the convenient from the meaningful. It's hard to get a dopamine rush just from *reality*. It takes a lot of effort, things like:

Working out

Flirting with an attractive person

Securing a promotion in your career

Eating a healthy meal

---

[32] Jelena Zorn, Gordana Arsić-Komljenović, Dragana Kastratović, and Marija Mladenović, "The Impact of Pornography on Children's and Youth's Mental Health: A Narrative Review," *Children* 10, no. 6 (2023)

Unhealthy sources of this same dopamine rush can come from things like:

Being a couch potato

Consuming pornography

Taking shortcuts on hard tasks

Eating junk food

Children are small humans who cannot distinguish between healthy and unhealthy sources of pleasure. If you condition them to seek the unhealthy sources – convenience – you will mar them towards shortcuts for the rest of their life. Is reality ever going to make them happy?

It's *convenient* to give your kid an iPad to get them to be quiet for a bit...

It's *convenient* to give them fast food rather than struggle with them over eating healthy food...

It's *convenient* to sit them in front of YouTube rather than running on the beach with them...

One question destroys these excuses: **Which is better for my children, not for my convenience?**

My friend Dr. Jonathan Schoeff and I just recorded a podcast together. He shared a stat which showed that 73% of people are overweight or obese in the United States. Did you know that it's more rare now to have a six pack than it is to be in the top 1% of wealth in this country?[33]

Our future is our children.

We can create a better future *for* our children by living optimally today.

GENDER REASSIGNMENT IN MINORS

What is a parent's responsibility when their child says that they feel different from the sex they were assigned at birth?

This is a controversial topic, and I'm excited to talk with you about it because it's also one of the most important topics affecting parenting and its future today. Let's start with a general overview of this issue, and then we will examine it in regards to our children specifically.

Let's start with this: **You cannot change your gender.**

Gender transition doesn't really exist, in the sense that it *never* works. You can flood your system with the opposite gender's major hormones, but you cannot change your chromosomes or your binary ability to reproduce. I'm not talking about sexual preferences. I'm talking about what you physically are. You can only be one or the other:

---

[33] Overweight, Including Obesity, Affects 73.6 Percent of U.S. Adults," *FastStats*, Centers for Disease Control and Prevention, 2017–2018

Male or female.

When we are talking about biological sex, what's between our legs, this is very obvious. Even in cases of biological abnormalities, such as hermaphrodites, we recognize these as abnormalities because of the primary binary. The problem today is that biological sex is being confused with gender expression, the latter of which we are not recognizing for what it really is.

I'm talking about the vast panoply of other genders. Things like:

- **Nonbinary** – A broad modern term for anyone whose gender identity doesn't fit exclusively into "male" or "female."

- **Genderfluid** – Someone whose gender identity changes over time or depending on circumstances.

- **Agender** – People who identify as having no gender at all.

- **Bigender** – Identifying as two genders, either at the same time or switching between them.

- **Demiboy/Demigirl** – Someone who partially, but not fully, identifies as male or female.

- **Helicopter** – Just kidding!

All of these things are simply made up. They're societal constructs that, to me, *are all manifestations of underlying mental health issues.*

I don't have any problem saying that...

Now, if you feel different, if you were born a man and you feel like a woman, and you want to dress as a woman – I don't care. But you're never going to be a female. You're also never going to use the female bathroom at my office. Sorry, but no. Maybe that sounds insensitive — I don't care.

What I do care about is the facts of biology, the responsibility of medicine, and particularly the responsibility of parents of children who "feel" different from their assigned sex at birth.

Not only should children **never** be given a hormone treatment opposite to their sex/gender, but neither should adults be given gender reassignment therapies.

Here's the reason why, using myself as an example:

My chromosomes are **male.**

My brain chemistry is **male.**

My body functions and developed as **male.**

The 'oil in my car' is the male-dominant hormone, testosterone. If you take that testosterone away and fill me with estrogen and progesterone instead, I'm not going to turn into a woman. Rather, I'm going to start having severe mental health issues like depression, anxiety, and suicidal thoughts. Then I'll have to get on antipsychotics, antidepressants, and anti-anxiety medications. Then I'll have to deal with the side-effects of that, and I may end up committing suicide.

That's not me being dramatic. A recent UCLA study found that 42% of transgender adults have attempted suicide, 81% have considered suicide, and 56% have engaged in self-harm.[34]

This is not rocket science.
Men need **male hormones.**
Women need **female hormones.**

Use logic, not emotion. Use science, not societal pressure. It may seem like tolerance to tolerate sex-reassignment, but when almost 50% of those who receive reassignment regret it, and when 42% are committing suicide because of the symptoms that derive from it, *our tolerance is actually harm.*

Therefore, not only should these kinds of surgeries and therapies not be tolerated for our children, it should be illegal across the board. Gender reassignment surgeries and therapies, except in cases of the intersex (hermaphrodism), is malpractice. Doctors who practice these things should lose their license forever.

I say that with all confidence. You can put it on the front cover of this book!

---

[34] Ilona Csanyi, Jody L. Herman, and Kerith J. Conron, *Suicidality Among Transgender Adults: Findings From the U.S. Transgender Population Health Survey* (Los Angeles: The Williams Institute, UCLA School of Law, May 2022)

HEALTHY SOLUTIONS TO GENDER DYSPHORIA

I return now to my original question, how should a parent respond if their child says they feel *different* in terms of their gender?

Jeff Younger, a father in Texas, faced this issue.

Back in 2018, Jeff found himself in a custody battle with his ex-wife, Anne Georgulas, over their twin kids. Their son had been saying since the age of three that he was a girl, and by age five he had been diagnosed with gender dysphoria. His mother, Anne, called for their son to transition, changing his name, making him wear dresses, and live as a girl. Jeff didn't believe that his son was transgender at all.

At first, the courts gave them joint custody. Later, Anne got full custody, but the judge said neither parent could move forward with medical treatments like puberty blockers unless they both agreed. Jeff went public – social media posts, interviews, political allies – accusing Anne of trying to push their child into irreversible changes. His campaign drew support from big-name politicians. His ex-wife wouldn't let up. She was adamant about giving their young son gender reassignment surgery.

In 2022, Jeff tried to stop Anne from moving to California with the kids, especially since California had passed a "trans sanctuary" law. He lost that fight. Then in 2024, a California court gave Anne full custody and the authority to make medical decisions. His son could now be transitioned without his consent…

Why do I bring this up? Well, when I looked into this case further I found something very interesting.

In a recorded video, Jeff asks his son, "Who told you you were a girl?"

"Mommy did."

"Why did mommy tell you you were a girl?"

"Because I *like them*.", his son said.

Where do kids get the idea that they are not the gender they are born with? In most cases, they're being conditioned and fed this information, usually by parents or legal guardians, or they're influenced by their environment which is increasingly advocating (not just *accepting*) abnormal gender expressions. Our kids are being told that they have a choice to be what they are not.

It's a lie.

Gender reassignment is detrimental to health and antithetical to reality. Men and women are not the same. We are polar opposites in balance.

The healthy solution to a child with gender dysphoria is to:

1. Find out where they're getting the idea from.

2. Correct their misunderstanding.

3. If that doesn't work, check their hormone levels.

If you reach step three, the child likely has a hormone deficiency relative to their age. What would have happened if Jeff and Ann had given their young son testosterone therapy, if that was indeed the source of his dysphoria and not just an implanted idea? The boy would realize that he's a boy. He would come into himself mentally and physically and emotionally. He would be thriving.

If you're a transperson and you're reading this (and I applaud you if you have read this far), my takeaway and my message is *tough love*. Tough love is what's needed. Yes, you may feel that you're in the wrong body *now*, and I sympathize with that, but giving you hormone treatment to reverse your gender is a false promise. We should give you hormone treatment to *affirm* the gender that you actually are.

It's an **insanity** in our culture that a parent can irrevocably alter the course of their child's entire life based on their own warped idea that their child is not the gender they were born with. Hormone blockers and reassignment surgeries are deadly weapons. Doctors who offer them and parents who allow them are making deadly mistakes.

OTHER HARMFUL DRUGS FOR CHILDREN: BIRTH CONTROL & PCOS

The prevalence of synthetic hormones in our society today, particularly in birth control, is a major factor in almost all of our female fertility and hormone issues.

Women and girls are completely stopping their menstrual cycle and inundating their bodies with synthetic, man-made hormones. Often, this cycle begins at the first period. Conversations with the doctor/parent usually go something like this:

"Well, are you having bad cramps?"

"Yeah, I am."

"Oh, well, this is gonna help with that: birth control!"

Instead of accepting menstrual cycles and cramps as normal, we're choosing the path of convenience. It's not just a pill for every ill. It's now a pill for *every pain at all*.

PCOS is very often caused by birth control.[35]

Doctors hand it out like candy, and instead of teaching women how to understand their cycles, ovulation, or fertility windows, we drug them. That's family planning in America, just medicate the problem away.

But our conveniences are killing us. There are studies that show clear links between oral contraceptives and post-pill amenorrhea, disrupted ovulation, and hormone dysfunction that looks a lot like PCOS.[36] That's not empowerment. That's dependence. And if you look closely, a lot of the "solutions" we're offering our daughters are setting them up for long-term dysfunction.

What's the alternative? Real sex education, by parents, not by the school system or the internet. Advance sex education rooted in reality, not the degenerate, fringe nonsense that gets passed off as "comprehensive" today. Kids need to be taught what actually happens in their bodies: the consequences of sex, what it means to transition from a girl to a woman,

---

[35] Chung-Hoon Park et al., "Influence of Combined Oral Contraceptives on Polycystic Ovarian Morphology and Serum Anti-Müllerian Hormone Levels in PCOS," *Clinical and Experimental Reproductive Medicine* 46, no. 1 (2019)

[36] H. S. Jacobs, U. A. Knuth, M. G. R. Hull, and S. Franks, "Post-'Pill' Amenorrhoea—Cause or Coincidence?" *British Medical Journal* 2, no. 6092 (1977): 940–42

and how pregnancy works in real time. They need to know that there are certain times of the month where the likelihood of conception skyrockets, and that ovulation is a powerful biological rhythm they can track and understand. That's knowledge. That's power.

Parents have to step up. Too many are squeamish, afraid to have the hard conversations. But if you don't, the system will fill in the gaps, and that system will teach your kids that popping a pill is the answer to everything. We should be empowering our children to make their own informed decisions based on real talk, not fairy tales.

CHAPTER 8

The Future of Medicine

The future of medicine is hormone therapy. Why? Because standard medicine has gone awry. It's become corrupt, dogmatic, and overfocused on symptom *treatment* rather than symptom *prevention*. The future of medicine is prevention and holistic (mind-body) wellness; it's staving off disease and chronic illnesses before they happen; it's reversing aging and dramatically increasing our average lifespan.

UNCHARTED TERRITORIES IN HORMONE HEALTH

There are several emerging technologies, some of which I am personally developing through my businesses, which will be revolutionary for hormone therapy, and our overall health and wellness. I've outlined a few below!

BIOMARKER TRACKING

Imagine a wearable band that could track your hormone levels around the clock — showing you where your optimal should be, when you're falling short, and even pinpointing the root causes of those hormone cascades. Think of it like a glucose patch, continuously pulling real-time data from your blood flow. That's where medicine should be headed: away from guesswork and toward prevention. Continuous hormone monitoring could transform fertility diagnostics, menstrual cycle mapping, and personalized treatment plans. And the tech isn't far off. Right now, I wear a WHOOP band to monitor sleep, strain, stress, and heart health. But what if that same band could also run a continuous CBC — no needles required?

The insights would be **game-changing.**

Imagine a woman going through their 28-day menstrual cycle, able to see their hormone cascade in real time. If they're having fertility issues, this kind of data could help determine why they're not able to get pregnant. Some other uses could be:

1. **EARLY ILLNESS DETECTION AND IMMUNE RESPONSE TRACKING**

   Continuous white blood cell count, inflammatory markers, and hormone data could flag the earliest stages of infection, often before symptoms appear. This would allow for faster treatment, quarantine decisions, or lifestyle adjustments to prevent illness from progressing.

2. PRECISION ATHLETIC TRAINING AND RECOVERY OPTIMIZATION

Athletes could use their real-time cortisol, testosterone, and growth hormone levels to fine-tune training loads, rest periods, and nutrition. This could prevent overtraining, accelerate recovery, and optimize performance cycles for peak events.

3. CHRONIC CONDITION MANAGEMENT

Patients with autoimmune disorders, thyroid disease, or diabetes could track relevant biomarkers around the clock, spotting trends or triggers that worsen symptoms. Data could be shared directly with clinicians or an AI companion for instantaneous medication adjustments and lifestyle recom-mendations.

GENE-SPECIFIC HRT

Gene-specific hormone therapy is also already here. It's an emerging approach that uses advanced genetic and epigenetic testing to identify how your unique DNA influences hormone production, metabolism, and optimal balance. By analyzing specific genetic markers, alongside environmental and lifestyle factors, clinicians can create highly personalized hormone optimization plans tailored to your body's blueprint.

At our clinic, we already offer genetic and epigenetic testing to uncover potential predispositions that may impact your hormonal health. While the science is not yet perfected, and researchers are still determining which markers most accurately predict early hormone decline or individual optimal ranges, the possibilities are exciting. In the future, gene-specific hormone therapy could enable:

Early Intervention: Imagine knowing years in advance that your hormone profile is trending downward, not waiting until fatigue, brain fog, or weight gain hit you like a brick wall. Early intervention through continuous monitoring wouldn't just track decline, it would flag potential diseases and genetic proclivities long before they show up in your doctor's office. Hormone and genetic data can influence our own life plans. With the right information early, you can tailor your nutrition, training, supplementation, and daily habits to stack the deck in your favor. That's the future: prevention as a lifestyle protocol, not a reaction to crisis.

Precision Dosing: Determining exactly how much and what type of hormone your body needs for peak function.

Personalized Prevention: Reducing the risk of age-related disease by addressing imbalances before they cause damage.

Your personalized genetic map could guide your treatment and help to craft proactive strategies to extend your vitality, health span, and even your life span.

It's not perfected yet, and there are still limitations like:

- **Incomplete Marker Mapping** – We still don't know all the genetic indicators that predict early hormone decline, optimal baseline levels, or precise dosing needs.

- **Epigenetic Complexity** – Your gene expression is influenced by lifestyle, stress, and environment, so DNA results alone can't account for all variables.

- **Limited Clinical Data** – While early results are promising, large-scale, long-term studies proving safety and efficacy across diverse populations are still lacking.

- **Cost and Accessibility** – Advanced genetic testing and interpretation remain expensive and aren't yet widely available through mainstream healthcare.

However emerging technologies impact hormonal treatments, one thing is certain: As the benefits of hormone optimization become clearer and clearer to the public, the shortcomings of our current medical establishments will also become clear. People will start to wake up.

PUBLIC AWARENESS VS. MEDICAL ESTABLISHMENT

People are still very much bought in to the idea that doctors know everything. They say things like, "They're the professionals! I'm going to listen to them. Why are we going to listen to Tomo? He's not even a doctor!"

While it is true that I'm not a doctor, I did acquire an advanced HRT certification through World Link Medical. I'm the only non-medical person to ever complete this, and I'll probably be the last because I got in on a fluke!

My point is that you don't have to officially be a 'doctor' to be informed. In addition, doctors themselves need to be continuously educating themselves on the latest and most non-biased information out there. At *Aspire Rejuvenation*, our medical director, Dr. Joseph Clark, is constantly educating himself. In fact, he was also at that World Link Medical course with me.

There are many other doctors out there that understand this reality. I applaud every single one of them. However, people need to realize that there are also a lot of doctors who are lazy, who do not educate themselves further after college beyond their CMEs (Continuing Medical Education). Many doctors are not thinking outside the box simply because they're taught *not to* think outside the box.

Doctors will change for the better when the people, their patients, demand change. The people need to wake up first.

This issue has already gotten as bad as it could get. The whole planet went through the 2020 pandemic. Apart from a few Scandinavian countries, everyone was forced or convinced to wear masks, take vaccines, and socially distance. The COVID-19 vaccines were not adequately tested, were not adequately efficacious, and are still potentially deadly and harmful.[37] I don't care what side of the political aisle you are on, if you still trust Big Medicine and Big Pharma after the pandemic, then you're either misinformed or in outright denial of reality.

I'll put it very simply: Establishment medical training reinforces rigid treatment algorithms that are outdated, symp-

---

[37] Menegale, Federica, et al. "Evaluation of Waning of SARS-CoV-2 Vaccine–Induced Protection against Omicron Infection in the General Population: A Systematic Review and Meta-analysis." *JAMA Network Open* 6, no. 5 (2023)

tom-focused, and corrupted by 3rd party economic motives. The COVID-19 response, particularly in the U.S., exposed these systemic failures. The future of medicine then is not just distrust in these establishments, it's *demand for something better.*

Health is **not** rocket science.

Hormone and regenerative medicine therapies, and their future developments, offers us a simple solution: optimize your health first, treat it second.

What's the number one cause of death in the US? Heart disease. What's the central cause of heart disease? Being overweight and obese!

Solve for that first before you treat the overweight and obese with medication!

It's that simple.

CROSS-SPECIALTY INTEGRATION

Medicine today is also over-compartmentalized. There are a lot of gatekeepers and specialists who make education and treatment difficult to come by. Many of us have had to see several different specialists for one specific issue.

New technologies like AI are breaking down these information and specialty barriers. The future is a very holistic approach where you don't see a psychiatrist for psychiatry, or an endocrinologist for endocrinology, but rather you go to one place that looks at your whole body and mind and gives you the preventative treatment that you need.

Of course, specialists will always be needed to some extent. I'm not saying that we should replace endocrinologists or psychiatrists. There will always be a place for them when it comes to diseases and illnesses specific to their fields. However, the problem is that these specialists are automatically doing the *pill-for-every-ill* treatment and not thinking outside of the box of what they've been taught.

At my clinic, we want to work better with these specialists. We encourage psychiatrists to ask about hormones first, before prescribing antidepressants, etc. Psychiatrists should refer to a hormone clinic first, saying something like, "I'm sorry you're feeling depressed. But hey, how cool would it be if this is just a hormone issue?"

"But, doc, I thought I was mentally ill?"

"But it could just be your testosterone levels. Let's check that first, and if that's not it, then we can look more closely at your mental health."

That's a life-saving conversation right there! Before labeling someone mentally ill for the rest of their life, let's check all possible causes first.

This is what's called cross-specialty integration. At Aspire Rejuvenation, we are already doing this. One of our major modalities happens to be hormones, but we don't only ask our patients about their hormone issues like an endocrinologist would. Rather, we look at preventive and regenerative medicine and wellness as a total scope.

For example, one of the questions for the hormone quiz on our website is going to ask if you've had depression, anxiety, and a low sense of self for an extended period of time. Why? Because we know, and data shows, that mental health issues come with a declining hormone profile, especially the major sex hormones, which we talked about in the previous chapter.

When a man has low testosterone, he is highly likely to have depressive symptoms, anxiety, and could even have suicidal tendencies. He doesn't feel like himself. The car has no oil in it. It's so low that it's starting to destroy itself.

Your mind is a part of that engine. Psychiatry, endocrinology, regenerative and preventative medicine, even sociology; these are not separate things by any means. They go hand in hand. Why have these disciplines not accepted this basic fact?

It's because Big Pharma doesn't want them to!

It's because, unfortunately, there are a lot of people that are on antidepressants, antipsychotics, mood enhancers, and mood killers, all of which are very profitable to push and sell.

In contrast, if you were to name me a symptom, I could name you the hormone deficiency that's probably the problem. If you fix the deficiency, you're off the medication. Big Pharma doesn't want that, and doctors don't know any better. Here's a great chart that shows you a symptom you may be having, how to treat it with hormone therapy, and what Big Pharma medication it would eliminate, along with an estimate of what revenue this pill-for-every-ill brings in per year:

Note: These are illustrative examples. Any medication changes must be clinician-guided.

Symptom you name	Likely hormone issue (to evaluate)	Hormone therapy that may address root cause	Common "pill-for-every-ill" this could reduce (examples)	Est. annual revenue (latest available)
Persistent weight gain, central obesity, carb cravings	Insulin resistance; low testosterone (men); estrogen/progesterone imbalance (women)	Testosterone optimization (men), individualized menopausal HRT (women), lifestyle to improve insulin sensitivity	GLP-1 drugs for weight loss/diabetes (e.g., **Ozempic/Wegovy**)	**≈ $26B in 2024 combined Ozempic + Wegovy sales**. (Fortune)
Hot flashes/night sweats, mid-night awakenings, irritability (peri/menopause)	Low estradiol and/or progesterone	Bioidentical menopausal HRT (E2/Prog)	Non-hormonal vasomotor meds (e.g., **fezolinetant/Veozah**) and off-label SSRIs for vasomotor symptoms	**Veozah in-market sales trajectory ~ $150–$250M (company projection band).** (irwebcasting.com)
Low libido, erectile issues, low morning energy	Low testosterone	Testosterone optimization	ED drugs (PDE5 inhibitors: sildenafil/tadalafil market)	**ED drug market ≈ $3.3B (2023), growing ~9% CAGR.** (The Brainy Insights)
Brain fog, low mood, anhedonia around hormonal transitions	Low estrogen/progesterone (women); low T (men); thyroid to assess	Menopausal HRT / testosterone optimization; treat thyroid if indicated	Antidepressants (category)	**Global antidepressant market ≈ $15B (2020) → ~$18B by 2027 (proj.).** (Fortune Business Insights)
Bone loss/osteopenia in midlife	Low estrogen (women) / low testosterone (men)	Menopausal HRT / testosterone optimization (with bone-health plan)	Osteoporosis biologics (e.g., **Prolia/denosumab**)	**Prolia 2024 sales ≈ $5B+ (Amgen FY2024: $1.2B in Q4; +8% full-year growth).** (Amgen)

Aspire Rejuvenation is not a hormone clinic. It's not an endocrinology practice. It's not a psychiatry office. It's all of those things and more. We are a total scope wellness, preventive, and regenerative medicine clinic. This is what we do: We're going to make you well; we're going to help you function optimally, body and soul.

That's the **future** of medicine.

ECONOMICS, ETHICS, & THE HIPPOCRATIC OATH

Medicine is economics.

That's a great thing!

I don't run a socialized medicine clinic, nor will I ever. Socialized medicine doesn't work. Canada is a perfect example: Go try to get surgery in Canada and you'll be waiting eight to twelve months.[38] That being said, our current system is just as victimizing, just in a different way. I call it **Chronic Care Capitalism**.

This is a business model where medicine stops being about making you well and starts being about keeping you sick, just well enough to function, but never healthy enough to leave the system. It's the revolving door where you walk in with one problem, leave with a prescription, and come back six months later with two more. Every pill has a side effect, every side effect gets another pill, and the cycle keeps the cash flowing. It's

---

[38] Fraser Institute. *Waiting Your Turn: Wait Times for Health Care in Canada*, 2024 Report. Vancouver: Fraser Institute, 2024.

not health care, it's disease management for profit.

Socialized medicine is not the solution to this. Rather, capitalism is the solution to capitalism's problem. Have you ever heard the expression, 'vote with your wallet'?

That's what you do. Instead of paying your doctor $300–400 an hour to prescribe you, optimize your lifestyle first. If that doesn't work, optimize your hormones. The more people do this, the more the system will change. Doctors will have to adapt or die as people start to wake up. Doctors should start now before it's too late. They've already committed to this when they took **the Hippocratic Oath:**

"I swear to fulfill, to the best of my ability and judgment, this covenant:

I will respect the hard-won scientific gains of those physicians in whose steps I walk, and gladly share such knowledge as is mine with those who are to follow.

I will apply, for the benefit of the sick, all measures [that] are required, avoiding those twin traps of overtreatment and therapeutic nihilism.

I will remember that there is art to medicine as well as science, and that warmth, sympathy, and under-standing may *outweigh the surgeon's knife or the chemist's drug.*

I will not be ashamed to say "I know not," nor will I fail to call in my colleagues when the skills of another are needed for a patient's recovery.

I will respect the privacy of my patients, for their problems are not disclosed to me that the world may know. Most especially must I tread with care in matters of life and death. If it is given to me to save a life, all thanks. But it may also be within my power to take a life; this awesome responsibility must be faced with great humbleness and awareness of my own frailty. Above all, I must not play at God.

I will remember that I do not treat a fever chart, a cancerous growth, but a sick human being, whose illness may affect the person's family and economic stability. My responsibility includes these related problems, if I am to care adequately for the sick.

I will prevent disease whenever I can, for **prevention is preferable to cure**.

I will remember that I remain a member of society, with special obligations to all my fellow human beings, those sound of mind and body as well as the infirm.

If I do not violate this oath, may I enjoy life and art, respected while I live and remembered with affection thereafter. May I always act so as to preserve the finest traditions of my calling and may I long experience the joy of healing those who seek my help."[39]

I've placed in bold the significant section: *prevention is preferrable to cure.* While "violating the Hippocratic Oath" isn't written into our criminal code, many of its core principles are mirrored in legal standards for medical practice. Therefore,

---

[39] Lasagna, Louis. Hippocratic Oath – Modern Version. Tufts University School of Medicine, 1964. https://www.pbs.org/wgbh/nova/doctors/oath_modern.html.

if hormone deficiency is the root cause of many symptoms, and doctors are not advocating for hormone rejuvenation *before* prescribing for those symptoms, how is this upholding the Hippocratic Oath?

Trigger-happy doctors who prescribe pills without checking proper levels of hormones and lifestyle choices first, should be charged with malpractice. Practicing medicine like this, which happens every day all around the world, would be like doing surgery without an MRI or a CAT scan first. Would you want your doctor cutting into your shoulder and just guessing?

Hell no!

Why then **do we accept** the same shortcuts when it comes to our health?

REGENERATIVE MEDICINE: STEM CELLS, PEPTIDES, & EXOSOMES

Stem Cells – The body's "master cells" that can turn into many different types of tissue and help repair damage where it's needed most.

Peptides – Short chains of amino acids (the building blocks of protein) that act like signals in the body, telling it to make more of something, like hormones, collagen, or healing factors.

Exosomes – Tiny "messenger packages" released by cells that carry instructions and materials to other cells, telling them how to heal and regenerate.

STEM CELLS

Stem cell therapies have an exciting place in the future of hormone health. New data suggests that these cell-based therapies may not only repair sexual function and optimize overall body performance but also regenerate damaged tissue and restore the function of organs once thought beyond repair.

What's remarkable about stem cells in particular is that they're 'smart'. Stem cells are able to find things wrong with your body that you may not even be aware of yet. So, let's say you do a shoulder injection of stem cells because you have a shoulder problem, but you also unknowingly have liver damage. Your injection is not necessarily site specific. Those stem cells may travel to your liver instead and repair that first.

This is why Stem Cells are so exciting for preventative medicine, because they can treat things you would otherwise not even be aware of yet!

PEPTIDES

Peptides also have great efficacy when it comes to regulating and restoring hormones. For example, **HCG** (human chorionic gonadotropin) is what's called a *peptide hormone*. It functions as a signaling molecule in the body. In regenerative medicine, it's often used to stimulate testosterone production in men or support ovulation in women, because it mimics the action of the luteinizing hormone (**LH**).

Other peptides like **BPC-157** and **TB-500** are what we call *healing agonists*. They tell your body to heal certain things.

Think of them like text messages sent straight to your cells with the instructions, "Fix this now!" BPC-157, for example, can speed up the repair of muscles, tendons, and even parts of your digestive tract, while TB-500 helps with tissue regeneration and reduces inflammation.[40] Neither one of these peptides is a direct hormone booster, but by accelerating repair and recovery, they put your body in a better position to function at its peak, and when your body works better, your hormones follow.

Peptides are just naturally occurring chains of amino acids, so in most cases, peptide therapy is very safe. That said, it's not a free-for-all. There are situations where you need to be careful. For example, if you have certain cancers, you probably shouldn't take a peptide that's a growth hormone secretagogue, because increasing growth hormone might feed that cancer's growth. Big point here: *growth hormone and peptides do not cause cancer.* Saying they do is just wrong; the science doesn't support it. Could they make an existing cancer grow faster? Possibly. Is that proven? No. That's why my clinic always runs labs first and monitors you closely.

In fact, you can't even get a peptide from us until we see labs and you have a consultation, because we care. We care about your health. We don't want you to do something to damage yourself. If you're considering peptide therapy, do so cautiously and with a professional who cares enough to do all possible due diligence first.

---

[40] Staresinic, Matea, Ivan Petrovic, Srecko Novinscak, Ivan Jukic, and Predrag Sikiric. "Gastric Pentadecapeptide BPC 157 and the FAK-Paxillin Pathway: Gastrointestinal and Liver Healing." *Journal of Physiology and Pharmacology* 61, no. 5 (2010): 507–514

EXOSOMES

Picture these as tiny cellular data centers that store and deliver critical information, like repair instructions and raw materials, to other cells, telling them exactly how to heal, regenerate, and get back to optimal function. I do an exosome IV push every single month with 240 billion exosomes, flooding my system with them. These little data centers go all over my body, and then my body uses them to regenerate itself naturally.

Your body's a remarkable machine. We are miracles of science and biology. These emerging technologies already have an established place in regenerative medicine, and the future is bright. I hope you catch some of my burning optimism here!

AI & HORMONE HEALTH

AI is already advanced enough to do what most doctors can when evaluating labs, health markers, and anticipating health and wellness.

I submitted my own lab panel once to ChatGPT and prompted it to assess the results. It was 99% accurate to what our own Dr. Clark, who is extremely learned, would have determined. If AI can already match doctors at their own game, does that mean we don't need doctors?

No way!

But it does mean that doctors can start using AI as a tool to be more efficient, patient-oriented, and objective. Doctors still need to prescribe medication, and the doctor will also see things that AI can't see.

At Aspire Rejuvenation, we will be working to incorporate AI into our healthcare routines (which is kept proprietary for HIDAA protection), not to replace our doctors, but to help them do their job better, faster, and be able to give more personal attention to our patients. This will also lower our costs over time and make our treatments even more affordable and bespoke than they already are.

THE HORMONE CLINIC OF THE FUTURE

As I write this, I am investing in a new technology for lab work that will give a patient a full lab panel in just a few hours. What will this technology allow?

Picture yourself walking into a clinic and seeing a doctor immediately. After your consultation, a nurse draws your blood and takes you to lounge in a comfortable laid-back chair, with an IV drip, where you're watching your favorite movie. 90 minutes later, before you've even finished your IV bag, you have your follow-up consultation right there with your practitioner. They go over your full panel labs with you and answer every question. They offer you a prescription to optimize your health, and you finish your IV drip. Then, you walk right across the road to a pharmaceutical partner and get your medication right there, right away.

Guess what? We just solved 90% of medicine in 90 minutes. No more waiting rooms. No more 2-3 month out scheduling. No more pill for every ill.

The hormone clinic of the future is an ecosystem of efficient, effective, and comfortable whole health and wellness.

That's what I want Aspire Rejuvenation to be. Quick diagnostics and detailed care, able to fix people's problems without the torment of waiting or high costs. This is not convenient for convenience's sake. These are not short-cuts. This is *efficiency for efficacy's sake.*

This is optimization.

CHAPTER 9

Towards a More Ethical Health Care,

with Dr. Joseph Clark

This next chapter is from my friend Dr. Joseph Clark, the head medical director of Aspire Rejuvenation. With my editor, Joseph Lawrence, he talks about things like ethical practice, AI, and the future of medicine. You won't want to skip this chapter, *especially if you're a fellow medical practitioner.* So, without further ado, I give you Dr. Clark.

Q. Thank you for joining us, Dr. Clark. Why don't you tell us a little about yourself and your background, specifically, how you went from a career in emergency medicine to now specializing in regenerative and preventative medicine?

A. So, interestingly enough, I've been an emergency physician for the last twenty-five years. I started residency in 2000. What I continued to see ever since then was a general decline in how patients were taking care of themselves, even people who saw their doctor regularly and did everything they were told to do. They still weren't getting better and had a lot of medical issues. It seemed that we, as care providers, just kept adding more medication, throwing more pills at them.

In addition, I went through my own health journey. I noticed I was having symptoms that were suggestive of testosterone-related issues. I went to my own doctor at the time but quickly realized he didn't know what I was talking or asking about and had very little confidence about the subject of hormones. He was reluctant to prescribe treatment, even though my [hormone] levels were low. It took a little arm twisting to get what I needed, and even then, the treatment was completely subpar.

I quickly did not feel great. In fact, I felt even worse. That discouraged me, so I started looking at hormone optimization clinics. I acquired a position in one and quickly realized all the ways in which I could improve it, that this was a position I could be passionate in. I became acquainted with Tomo after hearing about all the remarkable work he was doing in Florida. I reached out to him about opening a new location for Aspire Rejuvenation, and we really hit it off. We put our patients first, and I think they appreciate that we truly look at things differently than most medicines today.

Most medical treatment today is based on a reactive-type model, meaning that when a patient has a problem, they are given a pill, a temporary solution to mitigate that problem, while not addressing root causes or considering future problems down the road. For Tomo and I, we want to treat that problem that's in front of us right now in terms of its root cause, irradicating that before derivative problems occur later on in the life of the patient.

Q. Thank you. I thought it was very interesting what you said about your personal journey towards regenerative medicine, because Tomo had a similar experience – hormone crash, inadequate doctors, then charting his own course to wellness – I'm curious, what was your first impression of Tomo?

A. Haha, Tomo is a lot of what I'm not, which is why we work so well together! My personality is such that I like to work regular hours and solve people's daily problems. I'm not extremely outgoing, someone that can approach a stranger and say, "Hey, I like that watch; tell me what you do to get that watch." That's all Tomo. That's why he is able to do the things that he does. Our dynamic works so well because we lean on each other's strengths, mine is in medical expertise and organization. We're the two sides of the coin that turned out to be a good match.

Q. Wonderful! Moving into the topic of medicine and its future now: Stem cells, exosomes, peptides, these are cutting edge technologies. What role do these things play in the future of medicine?

A. In the past, a lot of the things that we did as doctors were just accepted as dogmas. If your doctor said, "Hey, do this," you just did it. It's not like that now; there's more pushbacks and with that, cutting edge therapies like the ones you mentioned, are becoming mainstream and more and more and more patients are interested in them.

Being in the age of AI and information, patients have more access than ever. They are more inquisitive; they investigate things more; they ask more questions; they research more. That's a great thing.

In addition, Big Pharma has always had influence on how doctors prescribe patients. Doctors don't have a lot of time [to select new medications], and so Big Pharma curates those selections for doctors. It's literally a kind of wine and dining thing, where Pharma reps will take a doctor out to lunch or to a seminar and push a particular drug. Because of that, many doctors are not following the most up-to-date research on how things are affecting people.

Pharma can't capitalize monetarily on peptides and stem cells and exosomes, and so that's why these treatments are not being advocated for yet. Medicine is a business. We're in this unique middle period where on the one hand the patient has desire for more alternative treatments, and on the other side Pharma's not supporting those therapies because they haven't figured out how to make big money on them yet. Big Pharma can influence laws, the FDA, and the decisions of politicians, and that impacts how these things can be used. Peptides are very, very safe and have an enormous amount of potential to help people, but they still might have their use prohibited by the FDA because of these economic factors. Things may have to get worse before they get better.

However, the more patients know, research, and buy these alternative treatments, the more mainstream they'll become. It'll be very hard for future generations to prohibit their use, because they do show benefit. The better medicine always rises to the surface. The future of medicine will be more and more patient-progressive and patient-driven over the next 10 to 20 years.

Q. It seems like medicine nowadays is very over-compartmentalized. There's a specialist for everything. How can regenerative medicine integrate with all of these specialties, perhaps encouraging them towards a more holistic view of the body and patient wellbeing?

A. That's a good question. I think medicine in general is a dogma-driven profession. Many doctors that train their successors are telling them what they learned, which may be already outdated information.

As time goes on, we'll see more integration of specialties and more professionals that adopt a holistic approach or even a *regenerative* approach to medicine. There'll be less medication and more investigation of root causes. People are living longer than ever nowadays, and they won't want to live the last twenty years of their lives as invalids. The golden years should be golden! That means optimizing your levels so you do feel your best. That means having options to treat injuries and fractures and musculoskeletal injuries and etc. with alternative means.

A patient asked me yesterday, "Well, menopause has always been there… Why do you have to treat menopause? Why do you have to go on hormone therapy?"

"Well, you don't." I said. "People have not chosen hormone therapy for years and years and years. But the fact of the matter is, *if you don't*, you'll probably get early cardio-vascular disease, osteoporosis, and lose muscle tissue as you get older, and those years that you do live longer may not be great years… So, if you plan to live longer and you want to take the most out of that time, optimize for your best health now before aging catches up with you more and more."

Optimization gives you better health, better quality of life, better marriages, better relationships, better whatever. That's the perspective that most doctors are starting to realize, not *medicating* patients but *giving* them longer and more meaningful lives. Instead of treating type-II diabetes with medication, let's advocate for exercise and healthy dieting first.

You asked about psychiatry. That doesn't often come to mind when you think of holistic or regenerative medicine, but it should. If a psychiatrist sees a patient who has depression, and that patient also has obesity, why is the psychiatrist not putting that two and two together and saying, let's optimize your lifestyle before we prescribe depression medication?

More specialties will grasp this approach over time. Even in the last ten years, I've seen a big shift, from cardiologists and neurologists, to especially OBGYN doctors who are advocating for hormone replacement therapy in women. The tide is slowly starting to shift.

Q. Following that track, what is your critical view of the future of regenerative medicine in terms of its applicability for neurological conditions like Alzheimer's, Parkinsons, and TBI (Traumatic Brain Injury)?

A. Cautious optimism. It's still too early to say, but there's enormous potential in stem cell and exosome use for these kinds of conditions. It's a new type of therapy, so there haven't been enough human trials or studies yet. Restrictions have also been put in place that prevented this necessary research. Other countries, which are less restrictive, have a big head start over us here in the United States.

Whenever these kinds of treatments are brought up by the patient, we as care providers have to be realistic with them about the chances of success. We must be transparent about what we don't know. We should never overpromise, especially when they're in a very vulnerable state. It would be a tremendous gift to give our patients stem cell treatment to definitively heal and repair neurological function, and I think that from the limited data we have, there's a lot of promise.

Garnering more research will help us improve our techniques, become more accurate in our doses, and select better products for better outcomes. Personally, I've seen patients that have had stem cell injections and exosomal infusions who immediately acquire better wound healing, better recovery, lack of pain, and decreased inflammation. I've seen people cancel their knee replacement surgeries after just a few rounds of stem cell therapy. It's fantastic.

Big Pharma makes money on people being sick, and so, if we find ways to make people not sick very cost effectively, it's a multi-trillion-dollar industry that is affected. They have a lot of power. We must find a way to circumvent that power first.

Q. Continuing from that point, do you see AI as perhaps a solution to this problem, making research and information more available and efficient? Is AI primarily a good thing, and what would you offer as points of caution to your fellow practitioners regarding AI use?

A. Caution is key. We don't want to lose the human element in medicine. Patients see their doctor because they want to have someone they can confide in, trust in, and identify with. We need compassion and care. That being said, could AI predict the reading of an X-ray better than a radiologist?

Yeah, that's probably something which will happen one day. AI has enormous potential and enormous dangers. The right place for it now is in research and prediction. AI could predict outcomes in research studies in weeks/

days versus months/years. The acceleration of research becomes an accelerated development of new treatments.

It's a good tool for doctors because it's hard for doctors to know everything all at once. Picture a patient's treatment plan being run through AI first and then determined by doctors next. This would allow for AI to predict dangers before they're missed, while still being under human oversight. There are a lot of errors in medicine, sadly, which AI models can almost completely eradicate.

However, the concern I have is not with AI itself, but with how it's used. Doctors cannot rely on it for everything, especially their own critical thinking. Maybe doing the right thing for the patient, even though less cost effective, is something that AI doesn't think about, and doctors need to remain sagacious in order to catch errors like this. AI is a tool. It's important to use the tool and not let the tool use you.

Q. You mentioned earlier that when you first entered this field, it was filled with scams, false promises, and overcharges, and Tomo highlights the same concern in his book. Many still see terms like "stem cells" or "peptides" as empty promises or even scams. As regenerative medicine grows, what ethical and accessibility challenges need to be addressed to build trust and ensure responsible progress?

A. The thing is to ensure and maintain a good balance between business and patient care. At Aspire, we try to maintain profitability, but we don't allow profits to drive medical decision-making.

In medicine today, unfortunately that's not always the case. We are under Big Pharma's influence which is profit-driven rather than outcome-driven. The onus is on us as practitioners to maintain a stance where outcomes are going to drive our decision-making. If a stem cell or exosome product is going to make people healthier, feel better, and have a better outcome, then we should be doing it, regardless of what's more profitable.

A profit-driven model mistreats people. In contrast, keeping costs in line with what people can afford, where patients have access to information which is honest and transparent, is most important, and also ultimately better for the longevity of the industry. Scams are as bad for business as they are bad for people.

The biggest challenge is to ensure that patients who need these treatments can get them from the good actors in this industry, not the bad actors.

Q. Would you support creating a watchdog group in this space, perhaps by teaming up with other ethical clinics, or does something like that already exist? In other words, what is currently holding bad clinics accountable?

A. The clinics that do have good reputations are still fairly small in number, and so we kind of know who those bad players are to some degree. As I said before, patients are smart. They do their research before they come to us. So, thankfully we're seeing less exploitation in the field as the exploiters die out. That being said, I would not be opposed to having some degree of self-policing.

It's a slippery slope though because ultimately one or more groups will become more powerful and push out others that may have good contributions. So whatever is done must be done fairly, with some degree of ethics, like you said.

For the most part, physicians in this realm want to do the right thing and want to treat patients fairly. Since this is a new industry, there's huge potential for huge profitability which can cloud doctors' judgments. But as long as we're holding ourselves and each other accountable, we will be okay. As doctors, we're constantly looking for improvement, because [medicine] is a constantly evolving situation.

Q. Last question, if you were speaking to fellow doctors about the future, how would you describe the best-case scenario for patient care 20 years from now?

A. Yeah, that's a great question. Eventually, we'll move from the current model where we're in a reactive state of medicine to a proactive state of medicine, and we're already seeing that shift. It's a slow, slow-moving process, but people are trying to be more proactive with their health, with their diet, with their supplementation and with their physical activity.

Young people today know the generation before didn't take as good care of themselves as they could have, and so the young have a genuine interest in ensuring a healthy and happy longevity for themselves. For doctors, this starts at the medical school and training level. Medical schools must break out of dogma and be more evidence-based and evidence-driven, outside of the umbrella-like Big Pharma influence. Pharmaceuticals should be a tool, not a driving force. Doctors must retain their own autonomy rather than having business influence dictate their prescriptions and their critical thinking. The future is patient-first, not profit-first.

More and more physicians will gravitate to this over time. They're waking up to it already. While they may not be in the same position that I am where they can start their own clinics, they can raise awareness and think critically: "I've seen this degradation of health and medical care over the past 20 years, and I want to be part of the solution, not the problem."

PART III

CHAPTER 10

Turning Health into Wealth

Why do we pursue optimal health?

When we achieve that optimization we've worked so hard for, how do we use it properly?

We can easily fall into the trap of becoming healthy for its own sake, fixating on it, obsessing over *gains*. Part three of this book is dedicated to a more intelligent viewpoint. In these last three chapters, I'll show you how:

1. Health is for achieving wealth and excellence (whatever your path is).

2. Health is for cultivating happiness.

3. Health is for building a lasting legacy and impact.

Becoming optimal is about becoming wealthier, happier, a better parent, a better person for your community and, if you're a faith-based person, able to better fulfill your God-given mission to impact the world. If that sounds like something you want, keep on reading.

If that sounds like something you're already doing, great! But I want to push you to do more.

HEALTH IS THE REAL WEALTH

It doesn't matter if you're a billionaire – if you're sick, all that matters is getting well again.

When we are facing an illness, any illness, from the flu to heart disease, we very suddenly realize the value of our health. If you were terminally ill, God forbid, wouldn't you trade all your money and all your wealth, all your success, just to live longer with your loved ones? You would. I know I would.

It doesn't matter who you are, a tragic diagnosis can strike you in an instant. For example, when the great actor, Chris Hemsworth, did genetic testing, he discovered that he carries two copies of the APOE4 gene, which is a known risk factor for Alzheimer's. That tragedy led Chris to make a change. He decided to focus on spending more time with his family, improving his brain health, diet, and regular exercise, to delay or even prevent the onset of the disease.

What matters most to Chris?

It's not *The Avengers* or even his great character, Thor. It's his time. None of us know how much time we have. When our sense of the time we have gets cut short, we realize more fully what really matters.

This is why we optimize.

Ask yourself this: **What matters the most to me?**

Whatever your answer is to that question, your health is the essential by which you cherish, cultivate, and appreciate that most cherished thing.

We all know a loved one, or will know a loved one, that will face a tragic diagnosis at some point in their lives. That may even be ourselves. We are all going to die one day. This is not an excuse for pessimism or nihilism. Rather, it is a reason for optimism because it means that we all will be given the opportunity to appreciate that loved one more deeply when that moment comes.

Optimizing our own health, and encouraging our loved ones to do the same, expands the time we have with each other, allowing us to love and appreciate and edify each other for a longer time.

This is why we optimize.

If I'm correct in the idea that we only get one spin around this world, that we only get one life to live (and if I'm wrong about that, then that's f#cking exciting!) then I want to live it for as long as I possibly can. I want to enjoy it too. The best news? The door is **open** to you:

You can go on Operation Optimal for yourself. You can do this. It's right in your grasp. Choose an optimal life and live it day by day. The greatest wealth you will ever have is your health:

Multiply that wealth. **Start today.**

HEALTH IS FOR EXCELLENCE

I know what it's like to be in a high-stress environment on low-hormones (non-optimization), and I know what it's like to be in a high-stress environment on peak-hormones (optimization). When I was a police officer, if I couldn't think straight or act fast enough, I could get myself killed or worse, get somebody else killed. It behooved me to become optimal.

The same lesson is true in entrepreneurship, business, or whatever your profession is. Optimizing our bodies optimizes our minds. A healthy mind is essential to success.

I've had times in business where I neglected my health for the sake of business —missing sleep, stressing too much, skipping my gym routine, or having cheat days on my diet. And guess what? My performance mentally, physically, physio-logically, in my personal relationships, and *even in my business* — everything suffered for it.

It's a lie, one that I used to tell myself, that you *can't* be in the best physical shape possible while also building your business and becoming wealthy. I know better now. The truth is that *you can do both*, and one will make you better at the other. The reality is that being in the best physical shape possible, being optimal, keeping myself young and vibrant and hungry for more success is giving me the ability to keep building on that success.

My goal is to be a billionaire one day. In fact, I'm going to be a billionaire. Why do I know that? Because I know that me at my peak of performance is unstoppable.

I don't say this to flex or to be cheeky. I say this because you, whoever you are, have the same possibilities before you. Not all of us are meant for or even desire to be entrepreneurs. That's fine. But we all have a dream. Maybe being optimal for you means you become a better piano player, or a better tennis player, or a better parent. Whatever the trajectory of your optimal, the point is to become a better you.

The benefits to my businesses from my optimization have been incalculable. That success also came with a cost: I've had to spend less time with my family. As I said before, time is our greatest asset. So, how do we focus our time on what matters?

As I write this, I'm sitting on a yacht with my good friend Rob Moore, the renowned public speaker and author of *Money: Know More Make More Give More*, and *Life Leverage*.

When I asked this question to Rob, this is what he told me:

"The idea of time management is a complete farce, and it's funny that people think we can manage time. You can't. There's nothing you can manage about time. The only thing you can do is *free yourself from time*. We can free ourselves from distractions and the things that don't matter."

How do we do that? We use what's called a focusing agent. This is not caffeine, Red Bull, Adderall, or some other shortcut to energy. The best focusing agent in the world is:

An **optimal** and **healthy** body.

ENERGY & BANDWIDTH

Whatever you do, if you can't focus, you are a diminished version of yourself. There are certain times of the day where your focus is at its peak. So, how do we design our routines to give our highest focus to our most important tasks?

Everybody's body is different. Some of us are early birds. Some of us are night owls. Structure your day around your peak performance. I happen to perform best in the morning, just like a lot of people do. For me, the early (early early) morning is a time when I can truly use my focus and peak brain activity without distractions. I like to be up hours before the rest of the world. Rob Moore thinks the exact same way. That's why he and I click so much.

It's not enough to just have a good schedule, however. You also have to understand the difference between where your peak energy should and shouldn't go. As an example, here's a lesson I've learned from running my high-level businesses:

Never let a $5 task interfere with a $150,000 task.

Often, we bog ourselves down in minutia. This busyness is often a mask for our lazy business practices. It's the easy way out of high-level, more challenging activities. It's a shortcut. This happens all the time, no matter the task. Things like:

- Choosing junk food because it's 'cheaper' than healthy food!

- Choosing not to network for your business because 'I have so much to do!'

- Choosing not to write a song because 'I have to practice my scales!'

- Choosing to skip leg day because 'It's my turn to cook dinner tonight, and I'm too *busy*!'

If you're someone who's new to building a business, you can break out of this laziness mindset with a simple question:

WHAT IS AN HOUR OF MY TIME WORTH?

You can answer this question easily: Take your weekly income and divide it by the amount of hours you work for it. That's your hourly rate. Are you worth more or less than the number you see?

If it's less, then you're either underselling your value or spending too much time on low-level tasks. The solution isn't to work harder at the wrong things; it's to **raise the value of your time**. That might mean learning new skills, charging more for your services, or outsourcing tasks that don't move the needle. The goal is to shift your hours toward high-impact activities that grow your business and justify your higher rate.

Evaluate each of your daily tasks **analytically.**

I'll give you another example:

Currently, as I'm sitting on this yacht on the Croatian coast, I'm also moving houses back in the U.S. I'm able to do this because I have a new assistant, Alejandra. Moving is expensive. But it's even more expensive *to me* if I had to handle the logistics in person, because I would lose the opportunity that networking on this yacht provides. The bigger *expense* is not being on this yacht with 51 people who are high-level successful, including my friend, Rob Moore!

These are the economics of the successful. We think not in terms of dollars and cents, but of opportunity and impact. I traded a 5$ task for a $150,000 task.

$5 tasks are things like:
(more mundane and something everyone hates)

- Designing your own graphics

- Answering routine emails

- Troubleshooting tech problems

- Scheduling appointments

- Driving across town to pick something up

$150,000 tasks are things like:

- Pitching an investor

- Closing a client contract

- Building a scalable sales system

- Writing the copy for your flagship offer

- Speaking on a stage or podcast to hundreds of prospects

Most people have a mindset that says things like:

"I can't afford a chef or healthy, pre-made meals."

"I can't afford a personal assistant!"

"I can't afford... [x]"

My response to you is to **change the way you look at money and income**. Money and income is, in reality, simply the expressions of how we use our energy and time. Using your energy and time for higher-value tasks doesn't *cost more*, rather, it increases your available energy and time exponentially.

I understand that, if you're strapped for cash, you need to work. You need to do some menial tasks to build from zero. But in order to do more than just tread water, dedicate whatever spare energy and time you do have to the high level. I'll put it simply:

Sacrificing as much energy and time
as possible to high -level tasks is
how you become a high-level person.

If you don't have any energy or time to spare, or you need more than you have, increase your bandwidth by optimizing yourself.

OPTIMIZATION, NETWORKING, & SOCIAL CAPITAL

At some point in your life, whatever industry you're in, you will be ready to get in a room with other top performers. That's called networking, and it's a high-level task that you will need to have the courage to choose. Here's a few examples…

If you're a **pianist**, would you rather:

- Practice your scales or

- Network with Ludovico Einaudi

- If you're a **doctor**, would you rather:

- Spend three hours filling out insurance paperwork or

- Meet a hospital director who could open doors to a new practice

If you're a **real estate agent**, would you rather:

- Cold-call strangers all day or

- Tour a $5 million property with a motivated buyer

If you're an **author**, would you rather:

- Typeset your own manuscript or

- Have lunch with a top-choice publisher who can distribute your book worldwide

If you're a **small business owner**, would you rather:

- Run errands for office supplies or

- Pitch your services to a client who could double your revenue

Remember, our optimal selves should be our normal selves. We are habituated to underperforming. If I'm more successful than you by your own definition of success, it's simply because you haven't optimized your best you (yet).

OPTIMIZATION GIVES YOU PRESENCE

Top-level people have an aura, a charisma, that no one else has. If you've ever been in a room with someone like that, you know exactly what I'm talking about. So where does that intangible energy come from?

To answer that, let's look at the opposite. Picture two men with the same high-level income. One is overweight, lazy, and drinking too much, but he throws on a $20,000 Gucci suit hoping it covers the truth. It doesn't. He's still fat, lazy, and drunk. His testosterone is probably in the basement, his mental health is on the decline, and the money only makes the mask shinier.

Now compare him to another man who is dialed in, his hormones optimized, his body lean and strong, his energy clean. He walks in wearing Crocs, a paint-stained T-shirt, and dirty jeans, and guess what?

He's the one who commands the room.

Optimization, confidence, and top-tier charisma are not things that you can buy. You can't buy being in shape. You can't buy being healthy. All the hormone therapy in the world doesn't mean jack if you don't exercise, diet, and lean into the hurt and the hard.

Top-tier aura takes **top-tier effort.**

PROOF

As I've shown you in this book, I'm a living testament to what optimization is and can be. I've told you my story:

- I was overweight

- I was depressed

- I was circling the drain, almost bankrupt

Now, after optimizing:

- I'm making more money than I ever dreamed of

- I'm happier and more fulfilled than I've ever been

- My future for my family and legacy is bright

But this isn't about me. I, along with many others, am simply proof that optimization works. I've already laid out how to optimize everywhere in this book, my workbook, my optimization routine, and my weekly blog. You have the roadmap. Now you need to drive the car. If you're not tracking with me yet, I'm going to keep punching this info in your face until you start putting the pedal to the metal. There're seven basic steps to legacy:

1. Start with optimal health.

2. Optimal health will give an optimal mind.

3. An optimal mind will make you more money.

4. More money will bring success (however you define success).

5. Success garners happiness.

6. Your happiness builds your legacy: Family, business, art, education, excellence, etc.

7. Legacy means you lying on your death bed with a smile on your face, knowing you gave your life your all.

ACTION STEPS

1. **CALCULATE YOUR HOURLY VALUE**

   Write down your weekly income and divide it by the number of hours you work. Use this number as your benchmark for what tasks you should be doing and which ones you should delegate or cut out.

2. **AUDIT YOUR DAILY TASKS**

   For one full week, track how you spend every hour. At the end, mark which tasks are $5 tasks and which are $50,000+ tasks. Circle the ones you need to stop doing or outsource immediately.

3. **DESIGN A HEALTH-TO-WEALTH ROUTINE**

   Choose one daily health habit (sleep, nutrition, training, or recovery) and connect it directly to a business outcome. For example, "Optimizing my sleep increases my focus, which improves my sales calls." Reinforce the link between health and wealth.

4. **SCHEDULE HIGH-IMPACT NETWORKING**

   Commit to one weekly action that puts you in the room (or on the call) with someone at a higher level than you. This could be attending a mastermind, reaching out to a mentor, or pitching a big client. Optimize your energy so you can show up sharp.

CHAPTER 11

Optimizing for Happiness

Most people chase happiness through pleasure, money, or status, mistaking comfort for fulfillment, but that's hedonism. True happiness isn't found in possessions or temporary highs; it's built on *health*, both physical and mental. Without health, lasting happiness is impossible. Even those facing illness can find peace through acceptance and gratitude, yet they'd undoubtedly be happier without disease.

That's why we optimize now:
to strengthen the body, sharpen the mind,
and live fully before hardship comes.

STOICISM & HAPPINESS

If hedonism is the sickness of our culture. Stoicism is the cure. This philosophy redefines happiness not as pleasure, but as discipline, the alignment of mind, body, and spirit with purpose. Where hedonism chases the next high, Stoicism builds endurance and gratitude.

Marcus Aurelius, in *Meditations* (a book I've written a foreword for), taught: Master your emotions and focus on what you can control. The journey toward health and happiness is never linear; we plateau and relapse. If we lack the right mindset, we stay down.

We can't control external events, only our reactions. If a hurricane destroys my house, I can cry, or I can act. Stoicism means choosing strength, choosing to act.

When I built my first businesses, stress often broke me. I cried myself to sleep, couldn't afford food or gas, and barely kept my office open. But I pushed forward anyway. That's Stoicism, refusing to let outside chaos control your mind. Stress can kill. Control it before it controls you.

Try this morning prayer I wrote for myself:

"I understand that everything is my fault. I understand the power I hold through focused action. I am not and have never been a victim. I'm grateful for the challenges God has blessed me with. If I ask one thing, it's for patience and understanding so I may walk through adversity with a smile."

THE POWER OF SELF-TALK

Stoicism is a workout for your mind. How you talk to yourself determines whether you crumble or overcome. Dr. Joe Dispenza teaches that shifting our self-talk from negative to positive builds confidence and clarity.

Our words shape our reality. When told "You have cancer," one person thinks, I'm dying. Another thinks, I'm going to be healthy.

Which mindset leads to better outcomes?

You can literally make yourself sick by believing you will be. The mind convinces the body. But the reverse is also true; you can think yourself well. Control your thoughts before they control you.

We all hear that inner critic saying:

"I can't do this."

"I'm not good enough."

"I'm an imposter."

But you can choose the response:

"No, I can do this."

"No, I am enough."

"No, I am the real deal."

That's Stoicism in action: discipline over emotion.

CULTIVATING HAPPINESS WITH GRATITUDE

Gratitude is the simplest path to happiness. Yet many people say, "I don't have anything to be grateful for." Bullsh#t—you woke up today, didn't you?

Some mornings, gratitude comes easy; other mornings, it doesn't. But those are the days it matters most. When I feel down, I start with:

"I'm grateful I woke up."

Even if I don't feel it, I say it. Every new day is an opportunity to do more, see more, and become more.

I also use a gratitude jar, a simple vase where I drop three slips of paper each morning, each listing something I'm thankful for. Every Sunday, I read them all. Sometimes it's big things like business milestones, or sometimes it's small ones like "grateful that I can see." The point isn't what you write, but that you practice.

Gratitude transforms your perspective. When you look back on a week — or a year — filled with these moments, you realize how much you've grown, how strong you've become, and how good life really is.

CULTIVATING HAPPINESS BY LIVING AUTHENTICALLY

When I left law enforcement in 2018, I was burned out and miserable. After twelve years on the force, I felt lost. I joined a medical clinic but didn't know where it would lead. So, I took a cruise to Mexico to clear my head.

Even there, the weight of trauma followed me. On the third day, after too many mojitos, I broke down and said to my friends:

"Thank you for letting me be me. This is the first time in over a decade I've felt I could be myself."

That moment hit hard. I realized I'd been living as "cop Tomo." I'd worn the mask of what others expected. Gratitude toward my friends gave me clarity: I could finally be authentic.

Since then, I've made it my mission to live as myself, imperfectly, but honestly. When I told my friends, they said, "Bro, we love you." That was all I needed to hear.

No one else will transform you. You're the driver and the car. Take control and steer toward your optimal self. Your true friends will celebrate that version of you.

ACTION STEPS

1. START A GRATITUDE PRACTICE

Every morning, write down at least three things you are grateful for, no matter how simple. Keep them in a journal or a jar and review them weekly to remind yourself of your progress and blessings.

2. REFRAME YOUR SELF-TALK

When negative thoughts arise, acknowledge them, then immediately replace them with affirmations aligned with your values. For example, switch "I can't handle this" to "I am capable and resilient." Practice this daily until positive self-talk becomes automatic.

3. LIVE AUTHENTICALLY

Reflect on where you may be living according to others' expectations instead of your own. Journal about who you truly want to be and take one small step each week that aligns your actions with that authentic self.

CHAPTER 12

Optimize for Legacy

Legacy means something different to everyone, but to me it's simple: *impact.* It's the mark I leave behind through my family, my businesses, and the people I elevate. One of my greatest goals is to spark a new health revolution in America and the Middle East. *Operation Optimal* is part of that mission. Whether it lasts a century or a single lifetime, I live for impact because I believe in it. Legacy isn't about me; it's about what I give back to my community, culture, and world.

If you've ever imagined your funeral, you've glimpsed what legacy means. Who will be there? What will they say about you? What stories will they tell? These questions aren't morbid — they're mirrors that show how today's choices shape tomorrow's memory. No matter your age, every action adds to the story others will tell about you.

LEGACY THROUGH MENTORSHIP

At forty, I've entered my mentorship phase, and it's been humbling to see how many people now ask me for guidance. Every opportunity came from the proof I've lived: my business success, my consistency online, and my willingness to share what I've learned.

Mentorship arises naturally from **authenticity and presence.**

When you live with integrity, people recognize it and seek your guidance — not because you demand respect, but because you've earned it. True mentorship is less about giving advice and more about offering perspective, empathy, and example. It's the process of sharing your experience so others can navigate their own path with fewer mistakes and greater confidence. Every time you help someone grow, you reinforce your own discipline and purpose. In giving back, you sharpen your character and expand your legacy far beyond yourself.

LEGACY THROUGH CONSISTENCY

Legacy isn't built in moments but in repetition. Consistency is the key to everything worth doing: health, wealth, wisdom, and impact. You can't get fit without consistent training or succeed without consistent work. Legacy is no different. Define what you want to be remembered for, then live that definition daily. Even reading twenty pages a day for two years can make you an expert in your field. Legacy, like mastery, grows one step at a time.

If you think, "I don't care about being remembered," challenge that thought. It's often just fear of failure or feeling too far behind. Replace that narrative with honesty and action:

"I may have fallen short before, but this failure won't define me. Today, I'll make one person's life better."

Every act of good — large or small — builds your legacy. **Consistency and sincerity are what last.**

LEGACY THROUGH FAITH

For many, legacy connects to faith. Whatever your beliefs, faith shapes the *why* behind your actions, the eternal reason you do what you do. I was raised Catholic but have prayed in churches, mosques, synagogues, and temples. Each faith expresses humanity's search for meaning and order. To me, what matters most isn't the label, but the integrity you live by.

That means walking with honor. That means keeping my word. That means acting from gratitude. I don't pray for things anymore; I just say, "Thank you." That gratitude keeps me humble, focused, and aligned with my purpose. Whether you call it God, the universe, or energy, let your spiritual awareness guide how you treat people. Seek your own place of peace, whatever form that takes, and make it part of your daily optimization, body, mind, and spirit working together.

None of us know what comes next after this life, and that's what makes it an adventure worth living. Live yours with purpose, gratitude, and consistency.

That is how you build a **legacy that endures.**

ACTION STEPS

1. DEFINE YOUR LEGACY

Ask: What do I want to be remembered for? Who do I want to impact? Visualize your legacy and write down what success and remembrance mean to you.

2. LEAD BY EXAMPLE

Mentor someone who looks up to you. Share what you've learned, show up when it matters, and make consistency your proof.

3. LIVE WITH GRATITUDE AND HONOR

Practice daily gratitude, act with integrity, and stay aligned with your core values. Your legacy begins in how you treat people today.

It's My Fault

It's never too late to change. I hope that's clear by now. Your own *Operation Optimal* starts and ends with one person: you.

Every chapter in this book has pointed towards a single truth: **you are the solution to your own problem**. No doctor, pill, or quick fix can replace the mindset that everything in your life – your health, your wealth, your happiness — begins with *ownership*.

Here's the mindset I live by:

"Whatever happens to me, good or bad, is my fault."

Try that the next time life throws something hard your way:

"I lost my relationship... it's my fault."

"I got fired... it's my fault."

"I was diagnosed with type II diabetes...
it's my fault."

Now say it when something great happens:

"I bought my dream car... **it's my fault**."

"My business is thriving again... **it's my fault.**"

"I've trained hard and feel stronger than ever... **it's my fault**."

Ownership works both ways. The same radical accountability that forces you to face your failures also gives you credit for your victories. That's the power of this mindset. If it's your fault, that means it's in your hands to fix.

Even if I had one day left on this earth, I'd still live with the mindset that:

I have the **power** to create positive change.

I'm **responsible** for what happens to me.

Every obstacle is an **opportunity**
God has given me to grow.

No matter your age — 25, 60, or 85 — the door is still open. What matters isn't where you start; it's whether you decide to start at all.

Look at yourself in the mirror today and say:

"All my problems are my fault."

Then take one step, just one to start, towards fixing them. Go for a walk. Clean up your diet. Book a blood panel. Call the person you've been avoiding. Do something that moves your life forward.

You've read this book. You've seen the science, the stories, and the systems that work. Now it's time to act. Ownership without action is just guilt. Ownership with action is *transformation*.

If you're ready to take the next step, scan the QR code below and download your free **Health Optimization Guide**. It'll give you a simple, step-by-step plan to start optimizing your health today: body, mind, and spirit.

Because once you take ownership, everything becomes possible. And when your life starts to change for the better… You'll know exactly whose fault it is.

Yours.

REFERENCES

BarBend. "Ronnie Coleman's Heaviest Lifts Ever." *BarBend*. Accessed September 2025. https://barbend.com/ronnie-coleman-heaviest-lifts-ever.

Bradley, A. H. M., et al. "Stress and Mood Associations With Smartphone Use in Young Adults." *Psychiatry Research* (PMC), 2023.

Coleman, Ronnie. "Ronnie Coleman on His Only Regret: Not Doing More Reps with 800 Pounds." Interview by Muscle Mind Media. TikTok video, 1:00. April 13, 2022.

Fraser Institute. *Waiting Your Turn: Wait Times for Health Care in Canada, 2024 Report*. Vancouver: Fraser Institute, 2024.

Józwiak, M., et al. "Multifunctionality and Possible Medical Application of the Stable Gastric Peptide BPC 157 (Molecular Basis)." *Pharmaceuticals* 18, no. 2 (2025): 185. https://doi.org/10.3390/ph18020185.

Lasagna, Louis. *Hippocratic Oath – Modern Version*. Tufts University School of Medicine, 1964. https://www.pbs.org/wgbh/nova/doctors/oath_modern.html

Menegale, Federica, et al. "Evaluation of Waning of SARS-CoV-2 Vaccine–Induced Protection against Omicron Infection in the General Population: A Systematic Review and Meta-analysis." *JAMA Network Open* 6, no. 5 (2023): e2314198. https://doi.org/10.1001/jamanetworkopen.2023.14198.

Schoeff, Jonathan. Statistic quoted in podcast on overweight/obesity prevalence in the United States (personal communication, cited in text).

Staresinic, Matea, Ivan Petrovic, Srecko Novinscak, Ivan Jukic, and Predrag Sikiric. "Gastric Pentadecapeptide BPC 157 and the FAK-Paxillin Pathway: Gastrointestinal and Liver Healing." *Journal of Physiology and Pharmacology* 61, no. 5 (2010): 507–514.

Travison, Thomas G., et al. "A Population-Level Decline in Serum Testosterone Levels in American Men." *Journal of Clinical Endocrinology & Metabolism* 92, no. 1 (2007): 196–202. https://doi.org/10.1210/jc.2006-1375.

Zorn, Jelena, Gordana Arsić-Komljenović, Dragana Kastratović, and Marija Mladenović. "The Impact of Pornography on Children's and Youth's Mental Health: A Narrative Review." *Children* 10, no. 6 (2023).

* 9 7 9 8 9 9 5 7 1 5 1 0 8 *